Supportive Care and Midwifery

Supportive Care and Midwifery

ROSEMARY MANDER
MSc, PhD, RGN, SCM, MTD

**Blackwell
Science**

© 2001 by
Blackwell Science Ltd
Editorial Offices:
Osney Mead, Oxford OX2 0EL
25 John Street, London WC1N 2BS
23 Ainslie Place, Edinburgh EH3 6AJ
350 Main Street, Malden
    MA 02148 5018, USA
54 University Street, Carlton
    Victoria 3053, Australia
10, rue Casimir Delavigne
    75006 Paris, France

Other Editorial Offices:

Blackwell Wissenschafts-Verlag GmbH
Kurfürstendamm 57
10707 Berlin, Germany

Blackwell Science KK
MG Kodenmacho Building
7–10 Kodenmacho Nihombashi
Chuo-ku, Tokyo 104, Japan

Iowa State University Press
A Blackwell Science Company
2121 S. State Avenue
Ames, Iowa 50014-8300, USA

First published 2001

Set in 10/12.5pt Times
by DP Photosetting, Aylesbury, Bucks
Printed and bound in Great Britain by
MPG Books Ltd, Bodmin, Cornwall

DISTRIBUTORS

Marston Book Services Ltd
PO Box 269
Abingdon
Oxon OX14 4YN
(*Orders:* Tel: 01235 465500
              Fax: 01235 465555)

USA
  Blackwell Science, Inc.
  Commerce Place
  350 Main Street
  Malden, MA 02148 5018
  (*Orders:* Tel: 800 759 6102
                  781 388 8250
             Fax: 781 388 8255)

Canada
  Login Brothers Book Company
  324 Saulteaux Crescent
  Winnipeg, Manitoba R3J 3T2
  (*Orders:* Tel: 204 837-2987
                 Fax: 204 837-3116)

Australia
  Blackwell Science Pty Ltd
  54 University Street
  Carlton, Victoria 3053
  (*Orders:* Tel: 03 9347 0300
                  Fax: 02 9347 5001)

A catalogue record for this title is available
from the British Library

ISBN 0-632-05425-5

Library of Congress
Cataloging-in-Publication Data
Mander, Rosemary.
    Supportive care and midwifery/Rosemary
Mander.
        p. cm.
    Includes bibliographical references and index.
    ISBN 0-632-05425-5
    1. Midwifery.   2. Maternal health services.
3. Pregnant women—Care.   I. Title

RG950 .M346   2001
618.2—dc21   2001025254

For further information on
Blackwell Science, visit our website:
www.blackwell-science.com

Contents

Foreword

Both midwifery and social support are old ideas and practices with modern names. The custom of experienced women in the community helping other women to give birth has been a feature of childbirth throughout most of human history; the importance of supportive relationships with others has traditionally been recognised in a whole range of social institutions, including marriage, friendship and participation in many kinds of organisations, both formal and informal. In this book, Rosemary Mander accomplishes a very timely task in bringing together much of the relevant evidence from the two domains of research on midwifery and support. In a committed and scholarly work, she examines the historical and contemporary intersections and conflicts between the two themes, and shows how they have performed a kind of mutually confusing dance against the backdrop of increasing medical power and control.

Perhaps the greatest paradox of modern medicine is its addiction to the technological, surgical and other clinical interventions at the cost of ignoring the therapeutic benefits of social care. Human bodies are inhabited by human beings: the connections between mind, body and social context totally undermine the model of bodies as machines. Yet western medicine has built its empire largely on this asocial, mechanical view, ignoring evidence to the contrary, for example, the well-known 'placebo effect' which is treated as an inconvenient distraction when it comes to assembling evidence about competing medical therapies. There is now an enormous body of evidence that social support improves health and life-chances and this includes both support provided by health providers as well as by family, friends and local networks. Feeling cared for and about is probably the most potent and benign tonic there is.

Midwives stand in a pivotal place when it comes to this evidence about the health-promoting effects of social support precisely because their role has traditionally included supporting childbearing women as well as providing clinical care for them. As childbirth moved progressively from the social to the medical domain in the twentieth century, midwives found themselves in a very difficult position. While in some places they were removed from the set completely, in many others they were displaced from centre stage and expected to play understudy to intervention-hungry obstetricians. Childbirth became a battleground – not only of competing professional and economic interests, but more importantly of practices and values. The rights of childbearing women to information, choice and control had a walk-on part in all of this, but 'consumerism' in the childbirth field, as Rosemary Mander shows in this book, has always been more of a faith than a science.

One of the 'founding fathers' of social support and childbirth research, John Kennell, once remarked that if social support had been a drug marketed by a pharmaceutical company, the evidence as to its benefits and freedom from side-effects would have led to its widespread promotion and adoption (and huge profits for the pharmaceutical company). Herein lies a major problem. Because supportive care is cheap – involving no fancy technology and usually provided by women, the world's cheapest labourers – the danger is that it will be hailed as a low cost solution to all the current sicknesses of the maternity care industry. If this resulted in increased resources for midwifery, and much more attention being paid to the potential of midwives in all cultural contexts to provide effective and supportive care, the suspect politics and false economics might not matter very much. But in a situation in which midwifery in many countries remains a besieged occupation, we badly need a more evidence-based approach to evaluating the best way forward. Rosemary Mander's book should really help us on this path to better and more appropriate research and more informed and dispassionate policy-making. *Supportive Care and Midwifery* should be key reading for researchers, practitioners and policy-makers alike: childbearing women, still often left out of the picture, will find it quite fascinating to know how often their feelings about the need for support are grounded in science, and thus should – in a rational world – be given priority in maternity service planning.

Professor Ann Oakley
Director
Social Science Research Unit
Institute of Education
University of London

Acknowledgements

I would like to express my grateful thanks to those who have helped me in the preparation of this book. This applies particularly to Edwin van Teijlingen and Irene Tzepapadaki. To my colleagues, Sarah Baggaley and Dorothy Whyte, I am grateful for their encouragement to travel along certain roads. Maureen Abate provided useful advice about a different health care system.

I appreciate particularly the help of the midwives who spoke to me about their experience of caring for a woman who died.

My thanks go to Iain Abbot for showing me the meaning and the reality of support.

Introduction

In this introduction I welcome the opportunity to contemplate the big picture as it relates to support. I also outline some of the broad themes which underpin the approach I hope to expand on in this book. These themes are in no way unique to support or to childbearing. They are features of the human condition which are as old as childbearing itself, but which occur even more universally and over even longer time periods.

Chronicity

It is a commonplace observation that human life moves forward in a cyclical fashion. This is reflected in the words of a song from the 1960s, which are taken from an even older source:

> 'to every thing there is a season, and a time to every purpose under the heaven'.
> (Ecclesiastes 3:1)

This observation applies to many aspects of the human condition. Perhaps it applies most obviously to fashions such as clothing, which results in skirt lengths and trouser widths fluctuating. Some of us will be aware that the same styles reappear regularly.

How do popular songs, biblical utterances and fashions in clothing relate to the provision of support in childbearing situations? I would like to consider briefly how human knowledge, and the behaviour which may derive from it, also develops in a cyclical fashion. Knowledge is dynamic and arises from a multiplicity of sources. These include personal experience and research-based evidence, as well as tradition, intuition and rote learning. In the present context, however, there are two phenomena which I would like the reader to bear in mind.

The first is what may be termed the 'chronicity' of human behaviour. It may apply only marginally less to the provision of health care than it does to human apparel. Fashions in interventions, treatments and philosophies may disappear and re-emerge in as short a time span as one person's working life. But often the pattern will take longer to unfold. Examples in the wider field of health would include the current movement towards what is known euphemistically as 'care in the community'. The recent revival of the treatment of infected wounds by the application of leeches is another illness-related example.

Fads and fashions are also seen to come and go in the field of maternity care. These fashions may relate to aspects such as the woman's diet, to her alcohol intake, to the place of birth, to who is present at the birth, to the contact between the mother and baby, to the position in which she gives birth and to a host of other aspects of the woman's and her baby's care.

It is inevitable that certain forms of care or certain approaches may be out of fashion or even be denigrated for a while, only to be 'rediscovered'. Breast feeding is an excellent example of a practice which has been discouraged at different times by, among others, our medical colleagues (Palmer, 1993). The reasons for breast feeding's renaissance in the 1970s are complex, but they may relate to economic, social and political factors (Coates, 1999: 12). Whether mere fashion contributed in any way to this renaissance is difficult to assess. The much publicised breast feeding by certain celebrities may lead to the conclusion that it did. Eventually and inevitably breast feeding has been shown by the production of scientific and statistical evidence to carry benefits previously unheard of; these include protection of the baby against gastroenteritis, respiratory infections, otitis media, urinary tract infection, atopic disease and diabetes mellitus (MIDIRS, 1997). Thus, the scientific seal of approval has been awarded to this womanly art.

Perhaps it should come as no surprise when, in these circumstances, we hear voices saying that we always knew that breast feeding was superior to other forms of infant nutrition. It may be that it is the production of research evidence which renders this previously intuitive knowledge acceptable to a wide range of interested parties. In this respect the story of support in childbearing may be comparable with the rather varied history of breast feeding. The history of support in labour is rehearsed briefly by Tew (1995: 188), who reminds the reader of the 'historic function of the midwife [as being to give] continuous companionship and support'.

This mention of the supportive function of the midwife serves as a reminder that this may be one of the few functions of the midwife which is common to this heterogeneous occupational group. Worldwide, midwives vary hugely in their training, their status and their functioning; continuous companionship for the woman, however, is a universally shared characteristic. It relates crucially and fundamentally to the original meaning of the word 'midwife', which means 'with woman'.

Panacea

As well as the concept of what I have termed 'chronicity', there is a second phenomenon which may be contributing to the current recognition of the benefits of support in childbearing. This second phenomenon, well recognised among medical historians (Dickson, 1954), is the assumption that a new discovery, irrespective of the narrowness of its application, provides answers to a multiplicity of longstanding questions. Midwives will recognise this scenario in the causes of the condition usually known as pre-eclampsia, which has also provoked many such questions and the 'answers' have been found in a whole series of new revelations, a particularly disconcerting one being the 'toxaemias'. The observation has been made that the causes of this condition have tended to coincide with the development of medical knowledge. As in the present context, though, a new or rediscovered phenomenon may be credited as being invested with an almost infinitely wide range of beneficial powers. Thus, it may become widely regarded as a universally effective remedy or panacea.

In her book entitled *Panacea or Precious Bane*, Sarah Augusta Dickson traces the health benefits which have been attributed by physicians and others to one particular questionably therapeutic agent. This substance was reputed to clear asthma and catarrh, to facilitate healing, to reduce abscesses and sores, to resolve headaches, to cure diseases of the neck glands, to end convulsions and epilepsy and to remedy skin conditions and pains of the abdomen and heart (Dickson, 1954: 59). While the beneficial properties of this substance were first recognised by 'priests, travelers or historians and not doctors' (p. 59), it was our medical colleagues who 'soon took the lead' in proclaiming the blessings of this supposedly marvellous substance. It eventually became known as tobacco.

Thus, it may be that a multiplicity of benefits are now being claimed for the phenomenon which is known as support. As will be shown in this book, the current claims may be founded on better evidence than the claims of the sixteenth century advocates of what was then called the 'holy herb'. It is necessary for us to question, however, the basis of the rationale for the current claims as to the effectiveness of support; we must also scrutinise the recommendations which arise out of these claims. In the sixteenth century the evangelical recommendations for the health giving properties of tobacco led to a lucrative transatlantic trade from North America to Europe and beyond. Although the transport of the current agent is in the same direction, it remains to be seen whether any other comparable benefits accrue through the modern acceptance and application of support in childbearing.

Professionalisation

A concept closely related to the development of knowledge, is also germane to this book. Significant to various of the actors, it is professionalisation. In a classical account of the professions (Carr-Saunders & Wilson, 1933) the essential characteristics of an occupational group aspiring to professional status are defined. Carr-Saunders and Wilson emphasise the training required to become a professional; not unrelated is the acquisition of a specific 'technique' during this training. A further crucial characteristic of an occupational group striving for professional status is the need for a relevant association which serves to promote both the interests of its individual members and the profession as a whole, as well as to enforce standards. The development of its own unique knowledge base is a further essential characteristic of a profession (Freidson, 1970). Ideally this knowledge comprises authoritative research, which is applied consistently and conscientiously by the members of the profession. According to Freidson, however, the ultimate and only significant characteristic of a profession is its possession of power or control. This power is exerted over both the client and other less well-established occupational groups. Included in this power is self-control, by which he means the ability to control all aspects of the group's work and which operates at both an individual and an occupational level.

Terminology

Throughout this book I refer to the midwife or the lay carer or the support person as being of the female gender. This is not intended to exclude males who may provide this form of care.

Although this book is not aimed primarily at an academic readership, it is my intention to adopt certain conventions which are widely used among the academic community. One of these is precision in my use of words. The relaxed use of terminology may be acceptable in situations where all who are involved recognise this relaxed approach and, hopefully, the intended meaning of the terms. In this book such a relaxed approach is not feasible. A distinction which will emerge as significant is between health care workers in general and medical personnel. The term 'medical' is not infrequently used to include a wide range of health related problems, services and personnel. In this book, however, the term 'medical' is being used quite precisely. I use it only to indicate personnel with a medical qualification and the interventions which they either practise on the basis of that qualification or prescribe for others to implement.

The argument of the book

Support, like a number of other terms such as counselling and debriefing (Alexander, 1998), has become something of a 'buzz word' in maternity care. For this reason, if for no other, it deserves to be questioned and examined carefully. As with other agents, like those panaceas mentioned earlier, support may be at risk of becoming all things to all people. It is fundamentally important, therefore, that at the outset we should know what this phenomenon comprises – as well as what it does not. Thus, in Chapter 1 I contemplate the variety of meanings of support and attempt to organise a way of thinking to clarify their relationship to each other.

If we are to know what support comprises, examining the phenomenon *per se* fails to provide the complete picture. In order to gain an accurate perspective we need to stand back from the detail and take in the complete picture, that is the context in which support is offered to the childbearing woman. In the second chapter, therefore, I focus on the organisation of the provision of health care, which invariably includes maternity care. I argue that the health care system and the way that it developed and is organised inevitably informs, and may actually determine, the interaction between the childbearing woman and those who attend her. As well as identifying the issues which serve to distinguish the systems of health care and maternity care, I examine three examples of countries' health systems which illustrate these distinctions.

Having taken in the big picture in Chapter 2, in Chapter 3 I adjust the lens in order to focus on the need for and the nature of support as it is provided for the individual woman by her carer or carers. Beginning with the nature of stress in childbearing, I move on to examine specific interventions which may be supportive. This supportive care may be provided by the informal carers, such as partners, relatives and friends, or by the formal carers who comprise part of the health care system examined in Chapter 2.

In Chapter 4, because this book originates in the UK, I examine the role of the midwife in providing support and the various manifestations of the UK midwife. I consider the ways in which the supportiveness of her care is likely to be measured. Additionally, a range of phenomena which may influence her functioning are taken into account.

As I have mentioned, support is a topic which has been subjected to considerable research attention. In Chapter 5 I scrutinise the research evidence, which is mainly in the form of randomised controlled trials. I attempt to critically assess the strengths of this evidence and any limitations which may exist. In order to make this assessment, I focus mainly on the environment; first, this applies in broad terms to the environment of the research in terms of the local health care system. Second, the environment includes the nature of the situation in which the woman experiences support. Third, also included is the psychosocial environment, which comprises the woman's relationships with those who are near to her and who may be offering support.

Chapter 6 follows on from Chapter 5 by considering the relevance of the findings of the randomised controlled trials. This consideration again draws on the background of the various health care systems, which I analysed in Chapter 2, and examines closely the functioning of one particular support person. In this chapter, as well as an organisational orientation, I also consider the implications of the research findings and the resulting recommendations for those who are most directly involved – the woman and her professional attendants.

While my intention in this book is to concentrate on the support provided for the woman, as will be shown at an early stage, the supporter also benefits from and perhaps in turn needs support. In Chapter 7 I consider the carer and how she is or is not supported in her role of providing support to the childbearing woman. It is necessary to contemplate the effectiveness of the carer in these more or less supported circumstances.

In the final chapter, Chapter 8, I draw together the argument which has been developed and advanced in this book, by making comparisons with certain situations which may have been or are comparable. This chapter also provides an opportunity to attempt to look into the future and to anticipate the development of support in maternity care.

The questions which underpin the argument developed in this book relate to issues of culture, of research utilisation and of professional power. The question which ultimately emerges relates to the extent to which a novel system of maternity care is able to be transposed and can effectively supplant another which has been in existence in a different cultural setting on a long term basis. I further question the transposition of research findings, which are based on hard edged numerical and statistical data, without recourse to the personal and human implications of that transposition. Issues of professional power arise which relate to the organisation of maternity care in different countries. What also emerges, as well as the limited significance attached to the needs of the childbearing woman, is the way that professional and other occupational groups respond to threats to their power base and, effectively, to the livelihoods of the members of those groups.

Chapter 1
Making sense of support

The challenge that this chapter title presents may appear too simplistic to need a sentence, let alone a chapter. To some of us the meaning of social support is so obvious that it is not necessary even to put it into words. For others the words may be problematic but we certainly know support when it happens. In the absence of words to describe it, however, we may find ourselves with many different ideas about what support comprises and without any common understanding of its meaning. In this way support may cease to be of any practical value. For these reasons it may be helpful to attempt to make sense of what support is about.

In this chapter I seek, first of all, to consider the plethora of terms which have been used in the field of support, in an attempt to decide which are appropriate and which are redundant. Then I move on to examine the nature of support and the forms which it may take. This material is then related to support in health and in illness in fairly broad terms. Such a broad examination is necessary because, through this book, I aim to consider the role of support throughout the essentially healthy childbearing experience. Throughout this chapter the strengths and weaknesses of the research approaches are taken into account. This is important, not only for the material which is examined here, but also to assist understanding of the issues which will emerge in subsequent chapters.

Terminology

If we are to make sense of support, as this chapter intends, it is necessary first to understand the quagmire of words which surrounds this topic. Whereas different terms are ordinarily used to indicate different aspects of a phenomenon, this is not the case in support. All too often the meaning of terms is indicated by the context. Examples of this are found when the term 'support' is occasionally used without any qualifying adjective. An example may be found in the writing of Robertson (1997), whose inclusion of 'companionship' is the only indicator that the nature of the support is by a health care professional.

Occasionally the support is defined as 'psychological' (Elbourne *et al.*, 1989). Alternatively, psychological support may be considered in conjunction with the more frequently mentioned 'social support', to form 'psychosocial support'

(Wheatley, 1998). The researchers and authors who use these various terms tend not to explain why one is preferable to another, which leaves the reader to make her own assumptions. Invariably the subject under examination is the same, leading to the conclusion that these terms are interchangeable. A term which may be used virtually synonymously with psychosocial and social support, but which is sometimes used more specifically, is 'emotional support' (Thoits, 1982). This leads us on to consider the forms which support may take.

The nature of support

In the same way as I have described the terminology of support as a quagmire, its nature may be only marginally less opaque. As Oakley (1988) reminds the reader, support may comprise membership of an organisation such as a religious group, or may comprise having access to a confidante; she suggests that being supported and being married may be regarded as synonymous. Some may regard the possession or donation of material resources as a form of support. The complexity and variable significance of the practical and psychological components of support cause difficulty in describing it and may render the definition so broad as to be useless. The breadth of support is suggested in the explanation for its attraction offered by House and Kahn (1985: 84):

> 'It suggests an underlying common element in seemingly diverse phenomena and it captures something that all of us have experienced.'

Thus social support may be defined in terms of positive interpersonal transactions (Kahn & Antonucci, 1980), which are likely to involve one or more of the following aspects.

Emotional support

Emotional support is a marginally more specific term than simply support, as it has long been used to differentiate the help which is given from the more practical or 'instrumental' support. This seemingly simple distinction was made by Gottlieb (1978) following research into how support is viewed by people with no particular expertise in this area. This study suggested that behaviour which is 'emotionally sustaining' is the form of support which is most highly valued and comprises listening and demonstrating concern and intimacy. The other form of support which this research identified, and which Gottlieb found to be of secondary importance to the respondents, is 'problem solving'; clearly that is of a more practical nature. This apparently simple distinction between emotional and practical support has been endorsed and refined since Gottlieb's relatively early study.

Emotional support has been further defined in relation to its more long term or continuing nature if it is to be effective (Miller & Ray, 1994).Thus, this is a facet of support which is likely to be of interest to policy makers responsible for the organisation of maternity care. Emotional support has also been defined in terms of 'the provision of aid and security during times of stress that leads a person to believe he or she is cared for by others' (Cutrona & Russell, 1990: 22). That this definition does little to clarify the nature of this aspect of support will emerge during the course of this examination. This already confusing picture is further complicated by the definition of emotional support offered by Power *et al.* (1988) as comprising reassurance, intimacy, knowing that one is loved and the certainty that advice will be available if sought. The reciprocal nature of support in general and no less of emotional support is demonstrated by Langford and colleagues (1997); these researchers' account of emotional support adds this dimension of what they term 'mutuality' to their working definition of 'feeling cared for, esteemed and belonging'.

Instrumental support

Instrumental support, as mentioned already, has long been distinguished from the emotional forms. This more practical type of support has been known by a multiplicity of other names, being the 'aid' component of the triad recounted by Kahn and Antonucci (1980). Often referred to graphically as 'tangible support' or material aid, instrumental support may facilitate well-being through either lightening the load or allowing more leisure time for the supported person (Wills, 1985). Langford and colleagues' (1997) reminder that such aid may take the form of goods and/or services raises the issue of the balance or reciprocity between the supportive and the supported person. It is in response to this issue that the concept of a network of support assumes significance. Thus, rather than being a one way transaction, which arouses 'reluctance' (Wills, 1985), a culture or an ambience of instrumental support may be more acceptable.

It is becoming apparent that these broad definitions of support are leading us to the question of the extent to which these aspects of support are really distinct. In this way, although the support provided in a particular situation may be instrumental, it may additionally carry emotional or possibly informational support.

Informational support

Informational support, while appearing straightforward, is explained as quite different from the transfer of relatively neutral factual material. This aspect, along with affect and aid, forms the triad of support described by Kahn and Antonucci (1980).

The nature of the information is spelt out in Cobb's, albeit rather dated, definition (Cobb 1976):

'information leading the subject to believe that he is cared for and loved ...

esteemed and valued ... [and] that he belongs to a network of communication and mutual obligation'.

By using this definition informational support clearly becomes synonymous with psychosocial support. Thus, yet again, edges blur and our image of this phenomenon begins to cloud.

The chronicity of support once more becomes significant in the context of informational support. Although the definition given by Cutrona and Russell (1990: 22) may suggest otherwise, emotional support as mentioned above is a continuing phenomenon, as the effectiveness of informational support is determined by its timeliness (Miller & Ray, 1994). This requirement is amplified by Langford and colleagues (1997) who state that information-giving becomes supportive only if provided at a time of stress in order to facilitate problem solving.

Esteem support

Esteem support is a form of support which is regarded as separate by some researchers and authors, while for others it appears to be integral to those forms of support mentioned already. Wheatley (1998) suggests that a person may use support to bolster her own self-esteem, whereas Langford and colleagues (1997) are marginally more objective, simply stating that appraisal support assists self-evaluation and affirmation. Wills (1985) delineates esteem support by recounting the element of self-exposure which is required and the vulnerability which this is likely to engender. For this reason, esteem support is less frequently sought or provided than the other forms. The level of trust between the supported person and the supportive person must be exquisitely high, and Wills describes this form of support as only being likely between close family members and longstanding friends. He indicates that for esteem support to be effective some degree of unconditional positive regard is necessary.

Deconstructing support

Although I, like other writers, have attempted to tease out the various strands which combine to produce effective support, the value of this exercise may be called into question. Whether the strands which have been identified as separate really are different is difficult to assess. As I have mentioned already the distinction between esteem support and informational support is uncertain, as is the role of 'aid' which may act instrumentally and/or emotionally.

Further blurring is inevitable if we consider the meaning of the various forms of support to the supported person. Regardless of the benefits or otherwise, each of these forms of support carries with it the message of concern for another human being, that is, that another person is sufficiently interested in one's welfare to become involved in the situation. On these grounds it may be necessary to regard these distinctions as artificial tools which achieve little more than closer scrutiny of this complex phenomenon. Thus, in this book I use the terms 'support' and 'social support' interchangeably to indicate a largely emotional relationship which carries with it elements of practical aid as well as information and affirmation. These components all serve to enhance the individual's self-esteem and assist that person's ability to deal with a situation which may be potentially challenging.

How social support works

In order to come to some understanding of how support may act to benefit the supported person, it may be helpful to take a step back to consider the situations in which support becomes relevant.

Stress

Although these situations vary hugely in terms of their nature, the one feature that they share is that they are perceived by the individual as negatively stressful. While the concept of stress may be another which is too vague to be of value, it is widely agreed that, as the term is currently used, there is usually some challenging or unpleasant aspect involved in it (Lazarus, 1966).

These 'unpleasant' aspects were recognised by Selye (1936) in his seminal work on the physiological systems which serve to protect us from a wide range of threats which may damage our bodies. Selye identified that these physiological processes not only protect us and help us to restore the body's equilibrium, but that they may also under certain circumstances actually cause damage. McEwen (1998) discusses these processes in terms of 'allostasis' involving the autonomic nervous system, the cardiovascular and immunological systems and the hypo-thalmic-pituitary-adrenal axis. The penalty which the body pays for the frequent effective protection offered by allostasis is the long term over- or under-activity of the systems involved.

McEwen recounts the body's response to a stressful challenge in terms of two phases. The first is the switching on of the allostatic response, involving the nervous and endocrine systems and the release of catecholamines, which sets in train the complex series of adaptive physiological mechanisms. The second is the switching off of this response. Inactivation ordinarily happens after the stressful situation has been resolved and the body systems return to their base-line levels. Problems arise, however, if the inactivation is less than efficient and the result is the prolonged exposure of the body systems to catecholamines, giving rise to a wide range of variably pathological consequences.

The effect of social support on stress

There is general agreement that support acts to reduce stress, although the precise mechanism is still the source of some contention. Oakley (1992a: 38) lists three ways in which support may reduce or minimise either stress or the likelihood of stress. She maintains that it may:

(1)   Act as a buffer to stress
(2)   Make stress less likely
(3)   Facilitate recovery from a stressful situation.

Because stress involves a pathophysiological process the assumption may be made that support interferes with the later pathological stages. It may be necessary to consider, though, the possibility that support is effective during the earlier psychological and physiological stages of the stress response.

According to Sarason and colleagues (1990), the functionalist view of support is that the support provided must match the stress present. This view is manifested in two hypotheses of the effect of social support. The first is the 'main' or 'direct effect' model, which regards social support as effective and protective against stress at all times regardless of whether the support is actually operational at the time of the specific stressful experience. This hypothesis may be based on the individual's belief or knowledge of the availability of aid whenever it may become necessary and that this belief or knowledge provides a stable structure to the person's life (Cohen & Syme, 1985). Wheatley (1998) dismisses this direct effect hypothesis as irrelevant due to being out of date.

The other main functionalist hypothesis of the effect of social support has become known as the 'buffering hypothesis'. This hypothesis suggests that support is only effective when it is available at the time of the challenging experience, that is, it protects the person when she is actually under stress (Cobb, 1976). In this way the person with stronger specific support is better able to withstand the effects of potentially negative or otherwise challenging life events than the person who lacks such strong and appropriate support. Although the buffering hypothesis is widely accepted and there have been a multitude of studies into its effects, the relationship between social support and well-being is not strongly supported (Schwarzer & Leppin, 1990).

Our understanding of the role of social support has been moved forward from the less than totally satisfactory buffering hypothesis by the work of Spitzer and colleagues (1995). These researchers, working in a health care setting, found that social support does have a significant effect on stress and adaptation to a challenging life experience. Their research shows, though, that this effect was achieved through the mediating effect of the individual's control over her circumstances, rather than merely as a buffer as had been widely suggested previously.

These functionalist approaches to the operation of social support clearly provide valuable insights. They may not, however, provide us with the complete picture. Sarason and colleagues (1990) examined the influence of psychological phenomena on the effectiveness of social support. These researchers found that an individual's sense of being supported is the accumulation of a number of inter-related factors. They regard being supported as the product of the person's interpersonal relationships and the meanings which the person attaches to them.

This amalgam is due to the interaction of, first, the activities of the person's support network, second, the support which the person actually receives or reports and, third, her perceived support which is a reflection of what she perceives to be available. These researchers argue that it is perceived support, rather than actual support, which correlates most strongly and positively with measurable outcomes, such as health indicators. The work of Sarason and colleagues (1990) is derived largely from attachment theory (Callaghan & Morrissey, 1993), the link being based on the hypothesis that a positive experience of attachment in infancy will facilitate the subsequent formation of effective and sustaining relationships into and throughout adult life. Although attachment theory is attractive as an explanation of social support through the early foundation of social relationships, it carries the unavoidable problem that for ethical reasons it is quite unresearchable and, hence, lacking in authority (Callaghan & Morrissey, 1993).

Issues

That clarity is lacking in the terminology relating to support has been clearly demonstrated already in the first section of this chapter. The problem associated with defining what constitutes support is only aggravated by the tendency of researchers and authors to ignore the complexities of this topic, resulting in the topic being approached too simplistically (Hupcey, 1998). Some of these complexities relate to the significance of the perception of support and of the timing of support, which have also been mentioned earlier in this chapter. The complexity of support may be compounded by certain assumptions which surround it, such as that of certain phenomena being equated with support, such as social class or family or marriage (Callaghan & Morrissey, 1993: 204). These assumptions are dismissed as 'romanticism or myopia' by Oakley (1992a: 28). Some of these assumptions may be related to another, possibly connected, example – the problem of distinguishing life events from the changes in support with which they are associated, such as marriage, divorce or bereavement (Callaghan & Morrissey, 1993: 207). As these authors observe, establishing causality through research, such as controlled studies, would be ethically problematical at least or, more likely, impossible.

Who supports?

This brief consideration of these issues leads inevitably to thoughts of the person or people who are involved in the provision of support. The offering or withholding of support may be through someone in an established personal relationship with the recipient, as in the above examples. Although a stranger with no history of any attachment may be preferred in some situations, the supportive role of the 'significant other' has been found in a meta-analysis of 93 studies to be the strongest variable in reducing the effects of adversity (Schwarzer

& Leppin, 1990). If there is a pre-existing relationship, its presence is likely to influence, that is increase, the effectiveness of any support which is being offered. Clearly, though, if the personal relationship features a history of conflict, achieving effective support may be less than easy (Sarason *et al.*, 1990).

As well as such *inter*personal considerations, Sarason and colleagues' interactive cognitive view draws the reader's attention to the individual's *intra*personal history. By this term these researchers refer to the likelihood of the individual's past experiences of support or of non-support affecting that person's later perceptions of being effectively supported. The importance of this intrapersonal history is clearly related to Bowlby's widely accepted theory of attachment. Such a deep seated and long term characteristic may cause the perception of support to be sufficiently stable to constitute a personality variable; this is associated with Sarason and colleagues having shown that the perception of being supported correlates highly and positively with feelings of acceptance and of being valued.

Although support invariably involves people, as emphasised by the definition devised by Schumaker and Brownell (1984), 'an exchange of resources between at least two individuals', it is not merely the 'sum of the parts'. Crucial to the provision of effective support is the environment within which that support happens. In this context the environment has become known as the 'network', which serves as a vehicle to facilitate support. In order to distinguish the network from the support which it may engender, Langford and colleagues (1997: 97) explain the network in terms of it being the structure, whereas support comprises the process which is facilitated; they go on to warn, however, that a network *per se* may not be beneficial, as structure may exist without function. A further warning relates to the assumption which may be made, that in this situation bigger is better; like other assumptions relating to this topic this may not be the case. The rejection of this assumption was originally reported by Kahn and Antonucci (1980), who warned that a large network should not be equated with large amounts of or better support.

How does support affect those involved?

It is necessary to assume at this point, for the sake of argument, that support is just that, i.e. supportive. The provision of effective support inevitably carries with it certain other effects, which have various implications for those involved and which may be regarded as spin-offs or as side-effects. These possibly unintended effects have been related to the rationale for the provision of support, which may be regarded as less altruistic than is sometimes assumed. This rationale is summarised as social exchange theory, which has been defined as 'the exchange of mutually rewarding activities in which the receipt of rewards is contingent on favors returned' (Tilden & Gaylen, 1987: 12).

Thus, when social exchange theory is applied, there appears to be some implicit form of bargain or barter, as it becomes apparent that both the provider and the recipient are beneficiaries when support is provided (Langford *et al.*, 1997: 96). In this way, the provider's experience may serve to reinforce and encourage generous supportive actions (Hupcey, 1998: 1233).

On the other hand, the provision of support may also have a less positive aspect. For example, the recipient may need to exhibit certain characteristics in order to attract the support which she needs and/or seeks. Sarason and colleagues (1990) observe that this exhibition may be sufficiently stressful to the person involved that the costs may outweigh the benefits of the support which is forthcoming. It has been noted that the 'provider orientation' in research into support has resulted in the costs of acceptance remaining unmeasured (Hupcey, 1998: 1239). The personal costs of the benefits of support emerged in the work of Lackner and colleagues (1994). These researchers examined support through the experience of the recipient and found concern about the rationale for providing support. The patient-informants were anxious that they might have difficulty repaying the obligation or debt which accrued due to the provision of support.

While the social exchange theory mentioned above implies some degree of balance in the mutual benefits or reciprocity of social support, Hupcey (1998: 1234/5) considers the problems which are likely to arise if such reciprocity is not balanced. Such an imbalance may be associated with a person perceiving that she receives either more or less support than she provides. In the former situation the person feels inadequate and the generous support ceases to be effective. In the latter situation, Antonucci (1985) suggests that this imbalance imposes further demands on the person who is already under stress.

When is support not supportive?

Although we tend to think of support as being beneficial, it is possible that intended support may not be effective or may actually be counterproductive (Hupcey, 1998: 1234). These unintended negative effects may result from, for example, conflicts between a longstanding confrontational relationship and the short term attempts to help (Coyne & DeLongis, 1986). Alternatively, actions which are intended positively may be perceived negatively due to their being inadequately thought through and, hence, less than appropriate. The examples of negative support given by Hupcey (1998: 1234) feature cigarette smoking, such as a smoker being ordered to cease smoking by a well-meaning but thoughtless health adviser or a cigarette being offered by a smoker who is trying to calm a non-smoking friend's anxiety.

As noted by Leavy (1983), in the same way as the perception of support is as beneficial as actual support, the perception of not being supported negates any benefits of support.

Research

In this brief account of the nature of and issues associated with support and research into it, it has emerged that problem areas persist. These relate particularly to defining what is meant by support and what it comprises, as well as assessing the extent of this phenomenon. It may be argued that support is obviously 'a good thing' and those who examine it more closely are likely to realise that many benefits have been demonstrated, even in the absence of any clear understanding of precisely how these benefits accrue.

For many this 'black box' level of understanding will be sufficient for attempts to be made to provide support. But negative support, mentioned above, should serve as a warning to those who are well-meaning without being sufficiently knowledgeable. Thus, research continues to be necessary and attempts continue to be made to answer these outstanding questions, in order to be able to provide and teach others to provide effective support as and when necessary. In the meantime the research on one particular aspect of support continues to encourage researchers to resolve these crucial questions of identification and measurement in order to facilitate effective intervention. This aspect is support in relation to health interventions, which is relevant here both for that reason as well as for its relationship to the almost invariably healthy phenomenon which is childbearing.

Support and health

The challenges of support in general which have been discussed apply to support in a health context. These problems relate partly to the quantification of social support as observed by Langford and colleagues (1997):

> 'the set of dimensions used to define social support is inconsistent. In addition, few measurement tools have established reliability and validity.'

These challenges have done nothing to impede the widespread recommendation and implementation of support in health care systems. According to Oakley (1992a: 24), the reason for this largely inadequately supported acceptance relates more to dissatisfaction and disillusionment with the alternatives than with enthusiasm for or conviction of the likely effectiveness of support. She describes how the medical model has proved less than relevant to a general understanding of health and illness in the broad terms in which they are widely experienced. Thus, the weakness, irrelevance or inadequacy of the usual medical explanations have resulted in a search for alternative theoretical frameworks. This search has resulted in the adoption of many more or less orthodox health orientations. It may be suggested that social support is situated at the more orthodox end of the continuum.

Background

The original research on the health implications of social support was undertaken in the context of mental health (Durkheim, 1951). This ground-breaking epidemiological study showed that unmarried men and women are more likely to commit suicide than those who are married. Durkheim's work is at least partly responsible for the widespread assumption of the direct and exclusive link between support and marital status which has been mentioned earlier. Within this limitation Durkheim's original assertion of the possibly fatal nature of a lack of social support appears to be an overstatement of the case. More appropriately, Durkheim's study served the inestimable function of drawing attention to the fundamental importance of a person's integration into the social fabric to the achievement of mental health. Perhaps unsurprisingly, this aspect of health has continued to feature prominently in the support literature (Duck & Perlman, 1985; Gottlieb, 1981).

The focus of this knowledge on the effects of support on the more physical aspects of health originated with the Alameda County study in California in the 1960s (Berkman & Syme, 1979). These researchers were able to draw up a 'social network index' which featured four forms of social connection:

(1)   Marriage
(2)   Extended family contacts and close friends
(3)   Church group attachments
(4)   Other group attachments.

Involving almost 7000 men and women, this prospective research showed that over a nine year period the person with the lowest level of support experienced an age-adjusted mortality rate 2 to 4.5 times higher than the person with the highest level. This finding still applied when a range of influential factors were taken into account, such as original health status, socio-economic status, ethnic background, substance abuse, physical activity, obesity, life satisfaction and use of preventive health care services. The findings of this study suggest that social support has a cumulative effect, the result being that for certain diseases the mortality risk increases with each decrease in social connection.

The framework used in Tecumseh, Michigan to identify risk factors was less restricted (House *et al.*, 1982). These researchers also included attendance at spectator events and voluntary associations and classes. After other risk factors had been statistically controlled these three factors were found to be significantly protective for men. The Durham County study was able to move the investigation of social support in the direction of perceptions (Blazer, 1982). This study found an increased mortality risk where social support was perceived to be impaired.

The Alameda County study, and those that followed and endorsed and refined the findings, may be criticised on a number of grounds. The first criticism is of employing a correlational rather than an experimental design (Langford *et al.*, 1997). This criticism may not be entirely justified, though, in view of the ethical difficulties associated with other research designs (see section on stress earlier in this chapter). A second criticism has been directed at these studies on the grounds of their use of the blunt instrument of mortality as the outcome measure (Callaghan & Morrissey, 1993). This point may be linked with the third criticism, which questions the relevance of using survival as a proxy measure for health (Oakley, 1988).

Effects of social support on health

In spite of the limitations of the research on the topic, it has been suggested that the effect of support on health and the reduction of morbidity and mortality operates in one or more of three ways. First, support may have its effect through changing the person's thoughts, feelings and behaviour in order to promote a healthier general orientation (House *et al.*, 1988). Second, Antonovsky (1979) has suggested that support may benefit the person by giving her a greater meaning to her life. This 'sense of coherence' may resemble the 1960s concept of 'getting it together'. Third, support may act by encouraging and enabling the individual to avoid activities which may damage health. Thus, support may facilitate behaviour which is likely to lead her in the direction of a 'healthier' lifestyle (Umberson, 1987).

Unfortunately, these ideas are not easy to support through research and have not been either validated or refuted. This is due in part to the methodological problems mentioned already, but also to the difficulty in operationalising the concepts of health and healthy lifestyle (Callaghan & Morrissey, 1993).

These three attempts at explaining the impact of support on health share another common difficulty, which is their neglect of the effects of the support network (see the section on informational support earlier in this chapter, and Cobb, 1976). The role of the network, within the limitations mentioned earlier in the section 'Who supports?', has been suggested as both beneficial to the individual and having the potential to resolve some of the researcher's difficulties. Rather than relying on the notoriously unreliable perceptions of support, Oakley (1992a: 30) has suggested that network analysis, a quantitative instrument, may be a tool which has the potential to provide accurate insights into social support. This potential has been refined to provide what may be a more precise picture of this phenomenon. Positive correlations have been identified between the size of the individual's social network, that is the number of contacts that exist, and the person's physical health status (Orth-Gomer & Unden, 1987). On the other hand, the quality of those relationships has been linked with the person's emotional health status (Barrera, 1981).This division appears rather contrived and may serve to highlight a dichotomy which may be less than real in the context of health.

Adopting a broader and more suitable interpretation of health, Schumaker and Brownell (1984) were able to identify the health sustaining functions of support. Each of these functions is closely related to the forms of emotional support outlined earlier in this chapter. The first of these health sustaining functions comprises the gratification of the person's needs for affiliation, through which the membership of the peer group is confirmed through restating her acceptability. Maintaining and enhancing self-identity is the second function, whereby the group acts as a mirror which reflects the appropriateness of the person's role within the group. Thus, each person obtains feedback which may serve to endorse the part which she contributes. The third function is enhancement of self-esteem, which relates more to the individual's self perception as a member of the group. These three functions were identified as promoting emotional well-being, but it is necessary to question, yet again, the reality or artificiality of the distinction between emotional and physical health.

Socio-economic class effects

The link between social support and the individual's health is clearly apparent. The phenomenon which is widely thought to be associated with both, but which is less easily investigated, is socio-economic class. Ham (1992: 200) discusses the UK picture as demonstrated by the higher mortality rates among children and older people in the socio-economic groups which he refers to as 4 and 5. In comparison with their more affluent counterparts in socio-economic classes 1 and 2, the mortality rates are worse for all groups. Additionally, and despite falling mortality rates, the differentials between the most and least affluent are clearly increasing. Ham recognises the limitations of using mortality figures as a measure of health. He admits that other measures, such as those of morbidity, are problematical due to their reliance on self-reporting.

The problem of accessing morbidity data was overcome by Soobader and LeClere (1999) in Boston, USA. These researchers undertook a cross-sectional study using data from the National Health Interview Survey and used perceived health in order to measure morbidity. Unfortunately, the data are weakened by their narrow focus on white men of working age. In spite of this they support the picture presented by the UK mortality data already mentioned. The researchers are able to conclude that income inequality, by which they mean poverty, acts as a major determinant of perceived health status.

The links between these three phenomena, socio-economic class, health and social support, are confirmed by the research undertaken by Matthews and colleagues (1999). These researchers examined the availability of emotional support, such as from friends and family and from organisations, as well as practical support. The data indicate that those in the lower socio-economic classes (4 and 5) experience lower levels of support than their equivalents in the higher socio-economic classes (1 and 2). The class difference applies particularly to the provision of emotional support. These researchers also noted gender differences which result in men having lower support than women. The tentative suggestion is made that these data may endorse the association between social support and health.

Conclusion

It appears that there are a variety of factors which prevent us from making sense of support. These relate, first, to deciding by what name this phenomenon is to be known. Next, there is the difficulty of finding agreement on what constitutes support as well as the circumstances under which it is and is not beneficial. A major area of contention is how the recognised benefits of support actually happen and whether the mode of action really matters anyway. Finally, the potential to ensure that the appropriate form of support is provided to those who may benefit from it remains elusive. The material on the effect of support on health indicators leads us to consider in Chapter 2 the role of health care systems and in Chapter 3 the relevance of support during the childbearing process.

Chapter 2
Systems of health care and maternity care provision

It has been argued in the context of the reform of health systems that, like it or not, a philosophy is fundamental to the provision of health care (Seedhouse, 1995). Seedhouse goes on to show how the lack of an explicit philosophy causes problems when seeking to change or improve a local health care system. In this chapter I am suggesting that the philosophy of the health care system is crucial to the provision of, not only health care in general, but particularly maternity care.

Thus, the philosophy which is articulated by the political leaders and the spin doctors and which is operationalised by the bureaucrats and the apparatchiks is likely to affect the interaction between the childbearing woman and those who attend her. With this significance in mind, it is necessary to consider the issues which influence the provision of, first, the health care system and, second, the system of maternity care provision. This examination of these issues will facilitate our subsequent consideration of the possibility of the system, and hence the attendant, being in a position to provide effective support for the childbearing woman. Following on from examining these issues, I consider the extent to which, and how, the maternity services in three specific countries are in a position to provide effective support.

Issues in the organisation of health care

A problem which I have encountered when seeking to describe health care systems from my UK perspective at the beginning of the twenty-first century is that they have a tendency not to remain the same for very long. In the UK, the 1997 change of government was widely expected to herald the return to the previous steady state which predated the health reforms of the1980s. The reversion which is actually materialising, however, appears to be more evolutionary than revolutionary.

The UK, however, is not unique in experiencing these trials and tribulations. The three other countries which I am looking at for purposes of comparison, Canada, the USA and the Netherlands, have also undergone their own traumatic equivalent of the UK's Griffiths reforms (DHSS, 1983). With similarly varying degrees of implementation, these took the form of the Lalonde report (1974), the Clinton Plan (Neuffer, 1993) and the Dekker report (1987), respectively. What emerges from this is not just that the health care systems of the western hemisphere are in a state of flux, which may be partly associated with the role of health care as a political football, but also that this unsteady state also reflects the relative imperfection of and dissatisfaction with these systems for providing health care.

The way in which a country's health care system operates is influenced by a range of phenomena, such as geography and climate, as well as history. Despite these unalterable variables certain issues emerge as significant in fashioning or organising countries' health systems.

Regulation of the health system is usually assumed to comprise a series of norms and/or restrictions which are operated by the elected representatives in a democratic environment (Arvidsson, 1995: 65). The regulation, which is literally defined as the rules, may be written in the form of legislation or directives, or may even be unwritten.

The prime purpose of regulation, which is especially relevant in the present context, is to ensure stability of the system. This control, which is largely by the state, becomes more significant when there is some degree of self-regulation, such as when certain powerful occupational and professional groups are involved. It may be argued, however, that these powerful groups do not actually comprise a threat to regulation by the state. Rather, as Johnson (1995) suggests, the reverse may apply in that these powerful groups may actually serve to enhance the regulatory power exercised by the state.

Secondly, regulation may be used as a form of cost control, which becomes more important when public resources are involved. The degree of state regulation varies. At one extreme are the highly state regulated countries, such as Sweden or the UK, where the health care system has traditionally been planned and controlled centrally. At the opposite end of the continuum are countries, such as the USA or the Netherlands, where state intervention is less in the so-called 'planned markets'.

As well as regulation being used like a stick in an attempt to control health care costs, as I have suggested earlier markets may operate simultaneously. Thus, *competition* has been advocated, encouraged and introduced in many countries in an effort to achieve greater cost effectiveness. Maynard (1994) writes scathingly of the paltry knowledge base on which these assumptions and interventions are founded. He argues that competition in health care is inefficient, associated as it is with uncertainty and short term benefits. Maynard continues by stating that political constraints, which prevent the development of classical markets and permit only quasi markets, further impede efficiency. This analysis is summarised by contending that evidence of the success of competition is lacking, due to the absence of serious research to investigate it. Perhaps unsurprisingly Pauly (1988), writing from his north American perspective whence competition has been most vociferously advocated, adopts a more optimistic view of its benefits.

A phenomenon which may be hard to disentangle from the concept of competition in a market setting is that of *consumer choice*. While widely advocated in the form of rhetoric (Neuberger, 1990), the reality of choice may be more elusive. As Neuberger reminds us, knowledge is fundamental to real choice. There is uncertainty about whether the consumer knows enough or is given sufficient information by the professionals to permit genuine choices to be made. She contends (Neuberger, 1990: 22) that the choice which the rhetoric maintains is available to the consumer is likely, in reality, to be exerted by the professional on her behalf.

A requirement which underpins the consumer's choice of services and which is all too easily taken for granted is the person's *access* to the range of services available. Obviously this may apply in a geographical sense to the consumer whose mobility is limited or who lives in an area which is remote and/or poorly served with transport or communication facilities. What may not be so easily apparent are the systematic problems of access which may be inherent in health care provision (Paton, 1996: 323). This may apply to certain services being less easily available to certain sections of the community or populations. Access to scarce services may be limited by rationing through the use of waiting lists. Perhaps simultaneously certain gate-keepers may be given the power to permit or deny access to those seeking access. On an individual basis, the service may render itself inaccessible through its ethnic, linguistic or gender orientation. There may be certain groups, on the other hand, who are more adept at gaining access to sought-after services, and whose ability in this respect may be related to socio-economic status.

Access is likely to be affected for some by the *method of payment* (Levitt *et al.*, 1995: 270). While the payment of medical personnel seems to attract most attention in the literature (Ham *et al.*, 1990: 100), there are other 'out of pocket' payments which are required of patients and others, which also deserve attention. Such payments may be related to the method of financing the health care system or may operate independently. Levitt and colleagues (1995: 276–9) show us that, although western health care systems are funded to differing extents by taxation, social insurance and private insurance, all require out of pocket payments for certain items. These include items such as prescription medicines, 'hotel services' or dental treatment.

A concept which is linked with and yet distinct from those mentioned already is *equity*. While this term may be used merely to refer to individuals' access to services, it may also be interpreted more broadly to include health outcomes as well as inputs. For many the right to health is a fundamental ethical principle as expressed by the World Health Organisation (WHO, 1986):

'The enjoyment of the highest attainable standard of health is one of the fundamental rights of every human being ... Governments have a responsibility for the health of their peoples which can be fulfilled only by the provision of adequate health and social measures.'

Inevitably such broad definitions raise far more questions than they answer. I regard, however, the underlying ethical principle of fairness in health as unarguable. Unfortunately and like other ethical principles, equity is the subject of much lip service; in the form of distributive justice, though, it is all too often disregarded in the process of planning health care (Saltman, 1997).

Issues in the organisation of maternity care

It may be helpful to think in terms of maternity care occupying a bridging position astride two camps. Maternity care links health care provision in its broadest sense on the one hand with the intensely personal and profoundly culture-bound phenomenon which is childbearing. Thus, having outlined some general issues of health care provision and before moving in the direction of the individual caregiver's experience of attending the individual woman, it may be helpful to apply these broad issues to maternity care in general.

Regulation

The regulation of maternity care has largely been effected through the state control of the occupational groups who provide that care. I will consider, first, the context of regulation, next moving on to consider historical examples; last I will consider the benefits and costs to those involved at a non-clinical level.

The role of the state in the regulation of maternity care was the focus of an insightful qualitative study by Burtch (1994). This researcher used the momentous changes in the Canadian maternity care system in the 1980s as the context for his exploratory study. Following a snowball sampling technique, he conducted semi-structured interviews with nurse-midwives and also with 'community midwives', whose practice was illegal/alegal at the beginning of the research. Burtch's findings are optimistic for Canadian midwifery and he considers that his data permit conclusions endorsing the safety of midwifery practice. Of more concern are the questions which this research raises about the limited control which the individual childbearing woman or midwife is able to exercise when compared with the overwhelming power of the state.

Context

Regulation of maternity care may be applied at a number of different levels and with varying degrees of compulsion. The supra-national influences may operate to include a range of aspects of health care, such as the World Health Organisation's targets to achieve Health for All by the year 2000 (WHO, 1978). Alternatively, organisations may focus more precisely on certain issues for a particular client group, such as the WHO/UNICEF Baby Friendly Hospital Initiative (1989). Certain supra-national organisations may, because of concepts such as freedom of movement of qualified European Union citizens, be in a position to influence the education of those professionals. This may be operationalised through instruments such as the EEC (1980) Midwives Directives.

Inevitably in the context of regulation it is usual to think first of the national legislative process. Of particular interest and, as a result, well-researched and documented is the legislation which regulates the practice, education and registration of the UK midwife. The UK midwifery legislation was originally intended to protect the public from inappropriate midwifery practice. This legislation also proved to have the indirect effect of protecting the midwife from litigation due to practising outside or below currently accepted standards (Lewison, 1996). The midwives' legislation was originally enacted in 1902 in England and in 1915 in Scotland. The purpose was to protect vulnerable women from untrained and unscrupulous midwives who were practising in a totally independent setting. This legislation, however, proved to have other, additional implications.

One of these was that the control of entry into midwifery was taken out of the hands of the church, which had long been responsible for licensing midwives. This control was transferred to medical personnel through their over-representation on the statutory bodies, the Central Midwives Boards (CMBs). The debate preceding the enactment of this legislation in the closing years of the nineteenth century involved many competing factions with different axes to grind (Robinson, 1990).

The medical practitioners were but one of these factions, and even they were divided among themselves. One group of medical practitioners considered that midwives should be registered because this would be one way of ensuring that they underwent at least a minimal training. Additionally, this would ensure that for even the poorest mother, in whom medical personnel had no financial interest, there would be a trained person to provide care. These medical practitioners were adamant that if any group controlled midwives it would be them. The other group of medical practitioners, among whom were many with a more general form of practice, perceived the possibility of a threat to their income. This group feared that registration of midwives, and giving them recognition, would raise midwives' status and increase competition for cases (Donnison, 1988; Robinson, 1990). The ninth bill and the first Midwives Act, in 1902, was carried largely in spite of the efforts of the General Medical Council. This legislation did however have widespread popular and parliamentary support and, most significantly, civil servants' support.

Interestingly there was nothing in the first Act requiring a midwife to be a member of the statutory body which it established although, as already mentioned, medical representatives were required. In fact midwives became members of the CMBs from the beginning, but only as representatives of other organisations, and certainly not to represent the midwife's professional organisation.

Another of the warring factions during the fracas preceding the successful passage of the ninth Midwives Bill was the nurses. They briefly occupied an important role, during which time they thought that the midwives might support their campaign for registration. The midwives spurned these advances on the grounds of being independent practitioners and having, in view of the current appalling mortality and morbidity rates, a more urgent need for registration. Thus rejected, the nurses came to oppose registration for midwives.

This situation of relative neutrality between nurses and midwives continued until the 1970s when new regulation was planned. This followed the recommendations of the Briggs report (1972) and took the form of the Nurses Midwives and Health Visitors Act 1979, which was implemented in 1983. The Act included a requirement that a midwifery committee should be established in each of the four countries and one with a UK wide remit. These committees were to be consulted on matters such as midwifery education and also have the function of considering any proposal to make, amend or revoke rules relating to midwifery practice. It may be that the 1979 legislation did little more than transfer the control of the midwife from the medical practitioner to the nurse. Thus, the need for a new Midwives Act is widely recognised (Symon, 1996).

As well as national and supra-national levels, regulation may also operate at an even more local level. This form of regulation emerges in the work of van Teijlingen (1994: 51) who mentions the local regulation of the municipal midwife in the Bavarian city of Regensburg as early as 1452. It is Marland (1993), though, who details the evolution of the municipal midwife in eighteenth century Holland. The context which Marland describes is one of the general decline of the European midwife due to limitations on her practice, her lower status and her difficulty in competing effectively. In towns such as Delfshaven, the local midwife found good support was forthcoming from the local authority. These town elders preferred to employ a midwife rather than a medical practitioner.

This arrangement clearly benefited both the midwife and the townspeople. The midwife was guaranteed a secure and not inconsiderable income, which carried with it a status at least comparable with the local traders. She was also excused the necessity of wasting time and effort competing with other midwives and medical practitioners for clients, which was a fact of life for those who did not hold such a favoured appointment. For the town authorities, there was the benefit of a midwife who would attend all the births within the town boundaries. The service which this midwife provided, they realised, would be of a good standard because of the frequent calls on her services and also because the town council were able to reprimand or discipline her should her standards fall below the level required.

History

As mentioned in the last section, the regulations in the Netherlands have long been supportive of certain groups of practitioners. This support operated on a local basis initially, but, more recently has become more wide-ranging. The result is that the provision of maternity care there is, in some ways, tightly regulated.

The state involvement in maternity care in the Netherlands has been traced back to the early post-Napoleonic era (van Teijlingen & van der Hulst, 1995). After being freed from France the country seemed to end up in an economic and cultural recession, partly associated with the industrial revolution in the Netherlands happening approximately a century later than in other European countries (van Teijlingen, 1994; 1999, pers. comm.). Hiddinga (1993: 45) suggested that:

> 'In general, this period of Dutch history is characterised by historians as one of uncertainty about the future of the new state. When the French occupation ceased in 1813, the Netherlands became stagnating and placid . . .'

This stagnation affected medical education particularly badly, although the precise reasons are uncertain. Schoon (1995) suggests that part of the problem may be attributable to the fact that Dutch universities, compared with their German counterparts, were focusing on teaching at the expense of research and innovation. This unfortunate situation may be illustrated by the way in which, until 1900, the textbooks which were in general circulation in Holland were mainly written in foreign languages. The most recent original Dutch textbook on obstetrics was dated 1817 and was still used in the latter half of the nineteenth century. It was not until obstetrics was recognised as an independent academic discipline in 1873 that the next Dutch language obstetrics textbook was published (van Teijlingen, 1999, pers. comm.). The sorry state of obstetrics is reflected in the following observation:

> 'Obstetrics in the Netherlands was in its infancy compared to abroad, the young age of the and the minimal experience of the first professors in obstetrics are evidence of that. The age of 28 and the inexperience of Simon Thomas led to serious objections being raised at his appointment in 1848.'
>
> (Schoon, 1995: 108, trans. by van Teijlingen)

Thus, the state was developing rapidly while the medical fraternity was seeking to organise itself; the regulatory context in which maternity care provided by the midwife evolved featured minimal competition from her medical colleagues. Part of this evolution comprised the Health Care Act 1818 which regulated a range of health care providers. This legislation applied to the midwife and to the medical practitioner equally and required all to take state examinations. Subsequently the state support for the midwife was further manifested in legislation enacted in 1865 which increased the requirements for medical education while recognising the midwife's official status. Additionally, fees paid to medical practitioners by clients were regulated at a higher level than those for the midwife, clearly providing her with a competitive edge (van Teijlingen, 1994).

The Dutch state in the twentieth century further favoured the status of the midwife. A regulatory framework was introduced to strengthen the position of the midwife in her power base in the family home. This was achieved through the recognition of the maternity home care assistant (MHCA), whose function is to undertake certain basic nursing and household duties around the time of the birth under the direction of the midwife. In 1926 the state legitimised the role of the MHCA, which is crucial to the Dutch midwife's high status. It is suggested by van

Teijlingen and van der Hulst (1995) that the inferior status of the MHCA automatically elevated that of the Dutch midwife. Simultaneously this 'low status' (van Teijlingen, 1994: 182) assistant performed the role which was crucial to the midwife in allowing the birth to remain in the woman's home.

In 1941 the regulatory concept known as *primaat* was introduced, which further benefited the midwife's position in relation to her medical colleagues. Under the Sick Fund Act 1941, the midwife's market share became virtually guaranteed by the requirement that the woman seeks the care of a midwife if there is one practising in her residential area. The sanction which was introduced under this legislation was that if the woman chooses to attend a general medical practitioner, the fees which are paid for maternity care are not reimbursed to her (van Teijlingen & van der Hulst, 1995: 181). Similarly, the fees of an obstetrician are only reimbursed to the woman if her childbearing experience becomes, or seriously threatens to become, complicated. In this way the role of the midwife as the expert in the care of the woman experiencing uncomplicated childbearing is protected by the legislation.

Thus, it is apparent that in historical terms the state regulation of maternity care in the Netherlands has been powerfully favourable to the midwife in comparison to the other providers of maternity care.

Politics

Apart from its party political connotations the term 'politics' is infrequently explained in spite of being widely used. This observation is exemplified in an otherwise admirable scrutiny of cross-national midwifery politics (Declerq, 1994). In the context of the regulation of systems of maternity care, I am using 'politics' in the more Machiavellian sense of 'astutely contriving or intriguing' (Macdonald, 1981). This form of politics has already been mentioned as having manifested itself in the 'fracas' which preceded the passage of the ninth Midwives Bill in 1902 to regulate the functioning of the midwife in England.

Another example of regulatory politics, which may be less well known because of its American context, is described in the work of Lubic (1979). This nurse-midwife recounts the attempts by the Maternity Center Association (MCA) to overcome the local and state-wide regulatory manoeuvring which threatened to impede the development of an innovative approach to maternity care. Lubic describes the MCA as a 'not for profit voluntary health agency' and it is widely recognised as one of the two longstanding organisations offering non-medical maternity services in the USA (Bourgeault & Fynes, 1997: 1053). In the early 1970s the MCA sought to introduce a 'childbearing centre' in the heart of New York City. The intention was to provide maternity care for families who were looking for care which did not involve hospital services and the inevitable 'invasive diagnostic and surgical techniques and machine technology' (Lubic, 1979: 3).

In her 'blow by blow' account of this confrontation, Lubic details how the regulatory framework was manipulated by the medical officials of the New York

City Health Department (NYCHD). She examines the role of the NYCHD commissioner in enforcing or waiving technical provisions of the city's health regulations. She suggests that the implementation or otherwise of these regulations results more from this person's strongly medical orientation and professional loyalty than from any health concerns (Lubic, 1979: 44). In a relatively early stage of this saga she gives examples of the regulators requiring confidential data on the activity of the childbearing centre. This is interpreted as the regulators seeking to extend their regulatory powers and thus limit the activities of practitioners beyond their sphere of influence (Lubic, 1979: 62).

At a later stage, the need for the MCA to provide services under the Medicaid scheme proved to be a major sticking point, crucial as Medicaid clients would be to the survival of the childbearing centre. The city officials gave 'violation of the City Health Code' as the reason for not permitting entry into the Medicaid scheme (Lubic, 1979: 65); thus health regulations were being used to impede this innovation. In response to this tactic the MCA were successful in raising the encounter to the level of the state regulations by enlisting the New York State Health Department. This strategy was successful in preventing the city regulators from interfering with the MCA offering maternity care. The sanction which achieved this outcome was the threat of state funding being withheld.

Following her account of the success of the movement to offer care in a childbearing centre, Lubic (1979: 94) is able to draw the conclusion that the regulations which control the availability of maternity services are manipulated in the same way as other human activities:

> 'Medical assemblages when confronted with conflict will use the same political tactics and maneuvers any other vested interest group brings to bear in order to maintain the status quo. Maintaining the status quo means keeping the seats and controls of power intact.'

Benefits and costs

In the course of this examination of the input of state regulation into the provision of maternity care, it has become apparent that there are a range of costs and benefits which may accrue to one or more of the participants in the childbearing scenario. The benefits of state support to the Dutch midwife have emerged clearly from the work of van Teijlingen and van der Hulst (1995). These researchers go on to compare the Dutch situation with that which applies more generally in the UK and refer to the 'general British dislike of government regulations and legislation on issues that can be regulated otherwise' (van Teijlingen, 1994: 181). This 'dislike' has been referred to as 'Anglo-American' (Larkin, 1994: 46), being commonly and perhaps stereotypically encountered among North Americans. It should not be assumed, however, that the existence of legislation supporting the practice of a certain group invariably has the effect of improving that group's status. The German midwife, for example, is protected to the extent that her presence is legally required at every birth; her status, however, is low even by general European standards (van Teijlingen & van der Hulst, 1995: 182).

The role of the state in supporting the continuation of home births has clearly carried certain benefits for the Dutch midwife. Home birth is an important example of community maternity care. It is also one aspect of an approach to care which is evidence of the desire for increasing effectiveness and efficiency commonly found among health systems (Ham *et al.*, 1990: 99). The paradox of community maternity care in the UK needs to be viewed, however, in organisational terms. While governmental policy favours care in the community in general, and the relative benefits of community midwifery have been extolled regularly in government reports, the numbers and proportion of home births in the UK remain low. This is due to the non-application of these policies to this specific situation (Selman & Haines, 1999: 108). The reasons for the failure to apply government policy in this particular context are beyond the scope of this book.

An example of the way in which governmental regulation may serve to benefit members of occupational and professional groups is recounted by Larkin (1994: 47); the principle, if not the extent, of this example may bear comparison with the regulatory favours extended to the Dutch midwife. Larkin details the statutory documentation required by the legislation at the time of certain life events. He argues that such notification or certification may serve to boost the group or individual professional status. He does not need to mention that under certain circumstances the income may also be boosted. What Larkin terms the 'medico-bureaucratic complex' may be extended far beyond simple documentation into more politically influential organisations, but such developments also extend beyond maternity care.

The functioning of the regulatory process also served to benefit the Canadian midwife, although the beginning of this process was, to say the least, ignominious. This was due to the *cause célèbre* following the death of a baby boy whose birth at home in Ontario in 1985 had been attended by a midwife. The inquest constituted an opportunity to bring into the public arena the practice of the midwife in Ontario. Both the medically dominated prosecution and the midwives' defence recognised the need for the regulation of midwifery practice, but how this was to be achieved was the source of contention (Bourgeault & Fynes, 1997). The jury recommended a compromise solution, consisting of, initially, the temporary regulation by the College of Nurses and, later, the development of midwifery self-regulation. The Health Professions Legislation Review appointed a provincial task force, which reported in 1987 that the desired route was self-regulation, discrete from both nurses and medical practitioners. The provincial government fully serviced the necessary developments to implement the task force proposals.

Bourgeault and Fynes (1997) consider that the strong provincial support for this ground-breaking Canadian initiative happened for two reasons. The major reason was the clear evidence produced to demonstrate the cost-effectiveness of midwifery care. Canada, like most countries, is keen to curtail its burgeoning health costs, and rationalisation by this route proved too enticing. The second reason is that the state was keen to be seen to be supporting women's rights and focusing on women's health issues. The midwife debate presented the government with an ideal opportunity to achieve this aim. In this way the 'woman friendly' credentials of the women Ministers of Health were established. The regulatory changes in Ontario began to be implemented in 1991 and were completed by 1994.

These changes may have been facilitated by the Canadian health care system's traditionally relatively large state input. This applies both to its role as the regulator of the health professions as well as to its financial responsibility for third party payment of medical services. The fiscal arguments, while not necessarily based on very strong evidence, may also be persuasive. The Canadian midwife may have taken advantage of this state involvement to advance her renaissance. This strategy bears comparison, though not favourably, with her co-professionals on the other side of the border in the USA. In order to achieve similar ends in a more decentralised health care system, the American midwife needed to enlist the support of her medical colleagues (Bourgeault & Fynes, 1997).

It may be that the experience of the midwife in Canada serves to endorse the possibly cynical observation made by an American political scientist (Declercq, 1994: 233). Focusing on politicians' and bureaucrats' power he spells out 'the two commodities that define their power: money and votes'. Because of the midwife's likelihood of rationalising care costs and her appeal to the women's vote she may, perhaps unknowingly, offer both.

Competition

At the level of the provider, competition within maternity care is probably no different from competition in any other field of health care. What we should consider here, additionally, is the likelihood of competition operating between the professional groups who are part of that provision.

Medical competition

The possibility of both inter-institutional and inter-professional competition is discussed by Ham and colleagues (1990). They consider that the 'ever increasing physician supply' (1990: 82) is leading to these professionals being required to compete to attract clients. The solution to this problem, according to these researchers, is that physicians are encouraging their clients to see more than one of their specialist colleagues during each treatment episode. This form of co-operation results in 'patient sharing' and the maintenance of medical incomes.

A slightly different form of medical competition emerges in DeVries and Barroso's (1997) forward-looking scrutiny of the role of the midwife. These authors recount the powerful role of the midwife as one of the two gatekeepers to the Dutch maternity services. This role provides her with not only the opportunity to encourage birth in a place which will facilitate the continuation of a strong midwifery power base, but also of controlling the access of medical specialists to her client, the childbearing woman. Thus, the midwife is in a position to exert sanctions which require medical personnel to compete in terms of their 'woman friendly' credentials in order to gain access to the client.

Midwifery competition

The situation of the Dutch midwife brokering competitive medical advances is perhaps unusual. The situation described by DeVries (1996: 171) of the midwife being in competition with the medical practitioner is more likely. In support of this argument, DeVries maintains that those occupational groups who are the greatest risk reducers are the ones to whom the highest status and the greatest power is attributed. He illustrates this point by referring to the formerly unrivalled power of the church, whose predominant place has now been usurped by the law and medicine. He suggests that the midwife may have done her professionalisation no favours by possibly having oversold herself as the carer of normality. If we accept DeVries' thesis of the significance of risk reduction, because of her focus on the healthy nature of childbearing, the midwife must always be assigned to a secondary status in relation to her medical colleagues. The obvious conclusion is that medical personnel are able to enhance their own status even though they may need to do this by creating risk by, as DeVries suggests, practising increasingly interventive obstetrics.

Competition with others

The limited ability of midwives to effectively counter medical competition has been demonstrated in a number of countries, including the USA and the Netherlands (DeVries & Barroso, 1997). The resources that midwives may utilise in this exercise are widely regarded as wasted. Competition with differing groups within the field of childbearing is particularly futile. Declercq (1994) demonstrates this point by drawing on the example of the poor professional progress of the American midwife in comparison with her colleagues in Canada. This sorry saga features the invidious, certainly counterproductive and well nigh fatal competition between the lay midwife and the Certified Nurse Midwife (CNM) (Bourgeault & Fynes, 1997: 1054).

This American example further illustrates the advantages of forming coalitions. These are evident in the longstanding supportive relationship between the CNM and her medical colleagues and the eventually mutually beneficial coalition between the CNM and her lay midwife sister. The formation of coalitions minimises the waste of resources required by competition. Declercq argues that such coalitions should be broadly inclusive to the extent of bringing in dissident practitioners; in this way, he maintains that conflict and/or competition may be kept and dealt with within the organisation. Examples of overcoming problems of competition in this way would include the formation of the Midwives Alliance of North America (MANA) and also the welcoming approach of the UK Royal College of Midwives (RCM) to the Association of Radical Midwives (ARMs). Declercq goes on to argue that the midwife should focus her opposition and utilise her resources against her competitors who pose a real threat through their ability to limit the practice of midwifery, rather than those who hold marginally differing beliefs about it.

Declercq, like others, recognises the medical practitioner as but one competitor in the maternity care arena. He argues that this competition may be the source of some disharmony, but that the threat exerted by other occupational groups should not be disregarded. The others who are mentioned by Declercq include the childbirth educator and the nurse. It is not impossible, though, that there may be others whose role also, and perhaps increasingly, impinges on that of the midwife. This scenario will be examined in detail in Chapter 6.

Consumer choice

The choices which are made available to the individual in the maternity area operate at an organisational level and at a clinical level. The consumer input into the organisation may be through political action, through local or community health councils or through single interest groups (Heginbotham, 1994). The single interest groups in this context include the campaigning organisations and pressure groups, such as the Maternity Alliance (MA), the National Childbirth Trust (NCT) or the Association for Improvements in the Maternity Services (AIMS). Edwards (1996) details how a campaigning organisation may be prevented from contributing to decisions about the future of maternity services by limiting the activities of its members. In her example the professional policy makers were more comfortable with the contribution of individual users of the maternity services than that of an organised pressure group.

The individual user's input at the level of the organisation has been defined as problematical, which is largely associated with the heterogeneity of the consumer population and the need of the organisation to streamline the service offered as far as possible by means of economies of scale (Havighurst *et al.*, 1988). Such findings are one of the factors which have impeded the development of a free market in health care in both the USA and the UK (Hunter, 1993; Mander, 1997).

It may be for similar reasons that choice at a clinical level, though much vaunted, is likely to be equally elusive. In some countries the 'package' of maternity care is explicit, such as that provided through a USA insurance scheme (Mander, 1997; Declercq, 1998: 852). The pressure on women and families to comply with such arrangements is powerful and widely discussed. In other maternity care systems the 'package' may be less explicit and may vary according to the locality and even according to the care giver involved (Garcia, 1999: 84). As Richards (1982) has argued so cogently, the choices available to the woman may relate to the fripperies of her childbearing experience rather than the fundamentals; the conclusion is that such choices are no choice. The woman's ability to take advantage of the choices which may or may not be presented to her is largely dependent on her knowledge base which, in turn, is dependent on the information she has been able to access. The problem of the uncertain existence of research-based information to facilitate the woman's choice has been addressed elsewhere (Mander, 1993).

Finance

As I mentioned in my introduction to this chapter, the methods by which health care is organised varies between countries, largely according to the philosophy of the policy-makers. Similarly, and also as mentioned previously, the methods of funding health care vary. One of the few factors which most health systems have in common is their dissatisfaction with the high level of spending on health care. This dissatisfaction is responsible in no small way for the epidemic of health system reforms which are being proposed throughout a number of industrialised countries (Paton, 1996: 308; Ham *et al.*, 1990). Much of the increase in health care costs is associated with demographic changes, in particular the ageing population. For this reason it may be assumed that maternity care is less likely to be affected by any financial stringencies. Perhaps unfortunately, the financing of health systems does not operate in this way. Some may argue that it is because the birth rate is at a relatively low level that maternity services are not spared their share of the economic pain. Again, we must bear in mind the cynical observation that the only phenomenon as important to politicians and bureaucrats as votes is money (Declercq, 1994).

It is a commonplace assumption that certain forms of maternity care are cheaper than others. These differences may be said to relate to the remuneration as well as the education, in terms of the duration and level, of the personnel involved (Bourgeault & Fynes, 1997: 1061). An alternative explanation for the differences in cost may be the status of the personnel or even the level of intervention which their practice carries with it and the iatrogenic problems which ensue.

The argument that nurse-midwifery is a more cost-effective way of providing maternity care has been utilised in different settings. In the USA, on the basis of work by Tom (1982), this argument was successfully advanced by nurse-midwives who were attempting to obtain recognition through third-party reimbursement from insurance agencies. In Canada the government used this argument because it was well suited to the rationalisation package which was that government's mainstay (Bourgeault & Fynes, 1997: 1054). In spite of these assumptions, what emerges from serious research is that the cost-effectiveness of such piecemeal approaches to providing maternity care is far from clear (Hundley *et al.*, 1995). Hundley goes on to argue that the costs of the introduction of midwife based maternity care into a medically dominated system are high and that this may have a deterrent effect on further attempts.

Medicalisation of maternity care

The increasing input of medical personnel and medical policies into uncomplicated childbearing is well recognised. These changes have been fully chronicled, including in the context of one particular intervention, by Graham (1997). The unbalanced power relationship between medical and other personnel which facilitated these changes affected the role of the midwife. This change is similar to the account of the technical nurse and the professional nurse at the time when the medicalisation of UK maternity care was in its infancy (Sheahan, 1972). More recently the power relationships have been likened to those of the various artistes who appear in a circus ring (Kirkham, 1986).

As well as these complex interpersonal and interprofessional developments in maternity care, practice has changed to become more interventive. Greater reliance on technology, combined with the increasing use of surgery and drugs, is associated with the medicalisation of maternity care. Helms and Bladen (1988) question the benefits of such interventive practice in general terms in a range of countries. These authors' misgivings about the excessive use of interventive technology are comparable with Neilson's (1999: 213) views on technology in maternity care in both developed and developing countries. His argument draws our attention to the dangers of the use of technology for reasons relating to prestige or fashion. The inappropriate use of technology leading to a requirement for its further use, particularly for defensive reasons, have been referred to as 'the technological fix' (Kaczorowski *et al.*, 1998). In maternity care, however, this vicious technological cycle has become recognised, in care in labour, as the 'cascade of intervention' (Varney Burst, 1983).

Neilson goes on to demonstrate that for many of the widely-used interventions, the evidence to support their use is either non-existent or equivocal. Cassandra-like, he warns that the attraction of the technological fix lies in the belief that such techniques provide an easy answer to problems whose causes are fundamentally complex. The problem is aggravated by the existence of such technology tending to require its use. Further, by investing in expensive and perhaps therapeutically unproven technology and interventions, scarce resources may be deflected away from 'lower tech' forms of care. These resource-starved services may be of established benefit, such as employing midwives or purchasing basic services such as cleaning.

The link between the organisation of maternity care and its medicalisation has given rise to concern in a number of ways. One example is the exponentially rising rates of surgical intervention, in the form of caesarean operations, in countries where maternity care is funded by insurance schemes. In their investigation of the changing, that is rising, caesarean rate in Latin America, Murray and Pradenas (1997) established this link. In the eight years from 1986 to 1994 the overall caesarean rate in Chile rose from 27.7% to 37.2%. This figure may appear unremarkable until it is examined more closely. Whereas the rate for women receiving maternity care under the national health scheme remained fairly static at around 28–29%, the rate for women using the private health insurance system rose to 59%. These researchers point out that the same medical personnel provide both types of care. The privately insured woman, however, is able to choose her obstetrician. It is suggested, therefore, that the insured woman is likely to have her caesarean operation planned for a time convenient to the obstetrician's shift pattern. On the basis of these findings, Murray and Pradenas warn that the organisation of health care is altered at our peril, as it may have a range of unforeseen, unforeseeable and unintended consequences.

Access and equity

Because the two ethical principles of access and equity are so frequently linked, probably because they impinge on each other so closely, I will consider them together in relation to their place in the maternity services. This close link is endorsed by the definition of equity which was used by the Resource Allocation Working Party (DHSS, 1976):

'equality of access to health care for those at equal risk'.

This definition gives the impression of being easily attainable. Unfortunately, this may not be the case as the thorny problems relating to resource allocation underpin equity or, rather, the inequity which is more clearly identifiable. The use of health statistics, that is mortality and morbidity figures, as indicators of the inequity of health care provision has become more and more refined since the Black Report eventually reached the public arena (Laughlin & Black, 1995). Through a series of publications the causal link between poverty and ill-health has been more firmly established (Ford *et al.*, 1994). In the field of maternity care, the perinatal mortality rate (PNMR) has long been used as an indicator of the inequity of access. This was demonstrated by a variation in one city's local authority wards of PNMRs between 8.5 and 37.9. These huge differences emerged in spite of the entire community being served by the same four units and community maternity services (McKee, 1984).

In maternity statistics the country of the mother's birth has been shown to be an appropriate proxy for disadvantage or 'social exclusion' (Schott & Henley, 1996: 38). In the UK this means that a mother who was born in Pakistan is twice as likely to give birth to a stillborn baby as her neighbour who was born in the UK. Similarly, the mother who was born in the New Commonwealth faces twice the risk of giving birth to a baby who dies in the neonatal period as her UK born friend. Attempts to overcome the inequity of provision which leads to such inequitable outcomes are fraught with ethical and political problems. The UK is one of the few countries which have attempted to overcome such disparities 'scientifically', albeit with limited success (Paton, 1996: 310).

For maternity care to be both accessible and equitable, Garcia and Campbell (1997: 16) maintain that there are a number of fundamental requirements. The first, which is becoming increasingly important with greater centralisation of services, is that the client, and her loved ones, should be able to afford to reach the place of care. Second, linguistic barriers are all too frequently recognised and 'solved' by either using family members or by drafting in staff with a knowledge of the language. These are far from ideal solutions as the family may have their own agendas and staff members may be less than sympathetic towards some of the woman's cultural needs. Third, there may be variation in the quality of care between providers or for categories of women within a particular provider unit. Fourth, certain forms of care may be regarded as luxuries rather than essential requirements. This might include, during the woman's post natal hospital stay, access to adequate suitable and clean bathroom facilities or, in a busy clinical setting, opportunities for talking to staff to unload an emotional burden.

The variable relationship between the budget and the service to clients leads to the question of whether equity applies merely to funding or whether the service 'on the ground' needs to be comparable. This debate is further complicated by considering the time span involved and whether short term care may need to be better resourced in order to achieve long term health benefits and, hence, financial savings. Such considerations may apply to improving access to maternity care through the possibility of home visits, the availability of drop in centres and satellite clinics, adequate interpreters and the development of special teams with a particular remit. Garcia and Campbell reflect on whether such outlay may be justified in the name of equity. They conclude that the problems of access and equity are largely unevaluated and that the associated moral decisions and political judgements urgently need to be subjected to wider debate.

Moderating effects

In considering some of the characteristics of health care in general and maternity care systems in particular, the role of politics has become apparent, less in the party political and more in the Machiavellian sense. The role of politics in the relationships between the actors in the maternity care scenario is scrutinised by Harcombe (1999). She considers the forms of power which are assumed or negotiated by the woman, the midwife and the obstetrician and the cultural background which influences the entire picture. The potential for real conflict concerning certain aspects of care, such as medicalisation, becomes clearly apparent. These political aspects are likely to at least moderate the health and maternity provision which is planned before it is actually implemented. Declercq (1994) makes recommendations about how less politically astute personnel may manoeuvre a path through this minefield; to do this he utilises a cross-national approach to analyse the political features of maternity care.

Further to the maternity system as planned being moderated by political influences, it is also likely to be changed by the behaviour of individual users. These changes may happen on the basis of group or cultural belief systems or on the basis of individuals' attitudes. Senden and colleagues (1988) show how cultural belief systems may affect the woman's use of certain services. These researchers investigated the labour pain expectations and labour pain medication use among women in Nijmegen (Netherlands) and Iowa City (USA). In a sample of 256 women, a large majority of the Dutch women (79.2%) did not use analgesic medication, whereas this applied to only 37.6% of the American women. The proportion in each group showing satisfaction with their pain control and the fulfilment of their expectations showed no significant difference. These authors conclude that the Dutch woman's behaviour and use of services is determined by a culture which convinces her of the likely successful functioning of her body. On the other hand, the woman in the USA is subject to a culture in which the medical model holds sway and influences her expectations and behaviour.

The findings of Senden and colleagues in relation to two cultures are endorsed by work by Howell-White (1997) on individuals' attitudes. This researcher found that the individual's belief system around birth and childbearing, and particularly her perception of risk, is likely to influence whether she chooses to be attended by a certified nurse-midwife or an obstetrician. Thus, individual beliefs also affect the woman's choice and utilisation of available maternity services.

Three systems of maternity care

In order to strengthen and further clarify the link between the organisation of the health care system and the support of the individual woman, I will now compare certain aspects of the maternity care provided in three western countries: Canada, the Netherlands and the USA. In the context of each of these countries I trace the way that the system of maternity care has facilitated or impeded the relationship between the woman and her carer.

In the course of this comparison, it is necessary to bear in mind the recent and ongoing changes in the health care systems which have been mentioned at the beginning of this chapter. These apply as much, and possibly more, in the field of maternity care. This dynamic situation varies over time, with changing allegiances and alliances, as well as between different geographical areas of one country, be they provinces or states. Of particular concern is a certain assumption which must be avoided: that because two neighbouring countries share a common border in a continental land mass, they share other characteristics in common. In my examination of two of the countries I show that this assumption is not justified.

Canada

Among the aboriginal peoples and early French immigrants to the area that later became Canada, the women cared for each other in childbearing (Relyea, 1992: 159). The customs which they carried with them usually involved some form of midwifery; I here define midwifery in its broadest sense as the woman being in the company of another woman during childbearing. It was under British rule in the late eighteenth century that the control of the midwife became established through certification in centres such as Quebec. By the end of the nineteenth century medical control of midwives was enforced by statute. Thereafter, competition between the two occupational groups resulted in the urban midwife's demise, due to her inability to withstand her medical colleagues' adverse propaganda.

In the more remote northern parts of the country, however, the situation was different. It has been observed that inhospitable terrain has the effect of discouraging medical practice. This deterrent action may be due either to the small number of clients, to their limited ability to pay or a combination of the two (Loudon, 1992). As a result 'outpost hospitals' were opened in the early twentieth century, staffed largely by nurses who provided comprehensive maternity care 'often without any formal training' in midwifery (Bourgeault & Fynes, 1997: 1056). It was mainly in this form that midwifery, though not called that, survived in Canada. Relyea (1992: 159) claims that:

> 'For many years Canada distinguished itself as the only industrialised nation which did not have legislation which supported midwifery practice.'

The resurgence of Canadian midwifery began with the 'counterculture' of the 1960s and 1970s and comprised lay midwives practising outside both the law and the formal health care system. According to Bourgeault and Fynes (1997: 1061), the timing of this resurgence is fundamental to the form in which Canadian midwifery eventually materialised. This is because this growth coincided with and was able to take advantage of the firm foundation which the women's movement had established in Canada. Through these powerful feminist influences, on both health care and the government, in some provinces the lay midwife became accepted, generally supported and eventually legal. This happy coincidence avoided the necessity for any medically-controlled or nursing-controlled compromise involving 'assimilationist' tactics to ensure survival. Such a fortunate outcome has been pessimistically summarised as 'a detour on the path to extinction' for the midwife (DeVries & Barroso, 1997: 253). The nurse-midwife did not have the opportunity to establish her power base in order to oppose the lay midwife; this meant that any competition from that quarter was effectively nipped in the bud through an alliance between the two groups of potential competitors.

The precisely fortunate timing of the Canadian development of midwifery applied also to the medical malpractice problems experienced first in the USA. The widespread opting out of obstetricians due to rising insurance premiums happened later in Canada (in the mid 1980s) than in the USA (in the early 1970s). This gave the midwife and nurse-midwife adequate time to cement their alliance before they needed to counter the competition for clients presented by the increased numbers of powerful general medical practitioners in Canada (Bourgeault & Fynes,1997: 1060).

As in the whole of north America, the emphasis of the Canadian health system is on institutionalised care (Ham *et al.*, 1990: 77). It is hardly surprising, therefore, that in their reaction against the standard medicalised maternity care, the feminist pioneers sought a form of care which also avoided institutionalised care. Thus, home birth attended by a lay midwife became the focal point which eventually secured legislation to foster a complete form of midwifery practice in certain provinces.

As mentioned already, developments in maternity care occur differentially. The result is that in the more conservative Canadian provinces little change in the organisation of care is discernible compared with the early twentieth century. A patchwork arrangement therefore appears in which complete and well-integrated midwifery care may be available in one locality, while in the neighbouring province, where medical power persists unchallenged, the woman may find that continuity of carer is seriously lacking. An example is where the woman is attended by her general practitioner until her pregnancy reaches 36 weeks, at which point an obstetrician becomes responsible for providing her care (Storr, 1999, pers. comm.). In a system in which continuity of *carer* is so grossly deficient, it is difficult to imagine that continuity of *care* is feasible.

The USA

The near total demise of the American midwife in the early to mid twentieth century may be explained in a number of ways. It may be attributed in general terms to the new immigrants endeavouring to adopt the characteristics of their new country. For this reason families became smaller (DeVries & Barroso, 1997: 252) and a more 'scientific' approach to care was sought (Jackson & Mander, 1995). The heterogeneity of American midwives was a second factor, which was due to the waves of immigration and the resulting variation among sections of the population and their care providers (Loudon, 1992). The immigrant midwife, who worked among her 'own people' in large centres such as New York City and Chicago, became part of a downward spiral of low expectations, low standards, decreasing numbers and low demand for services. In association with the eventual decline of large scale legal immigration, this midwife together with the rural midwife, who was usually a neighbour midwife, soon succumbed. The southern black midwife, however, managed to survive, along with two nurse-midwifery organisations. One of these organisations was mentioned earlier, the Maternity Center Association of New York City, and the other was the Frontier Nursing Service of Kentucky (Bourgeault & Fynes,1997: 1053).

In the 1960s, with the development of the movement that was called in the USA 'natural childbirth', the certified nurse-midwife (CNM) experienced an increased demand for her services. In order to achieve this, however, the close support, back-up or 'sponsorship' of a physician was essential (Bourgeault & Fynes, 1997: 1053; Mander, 1997). Because of this cosy relationship, the American nurse-midwife has been criticised by being called a 'physician extender' (DeVries & Barroso, 1997: 265).

The non-nurse-midwife in the USA is known by a variety of names, such as lay midwife or traditional midwife or direct entry midwife. Because the midwives who are known to me prefer the latter title, that is the one I use. The status of this midwife has for a long while been problematical, originally due to the illegal nature of her work and more recently due to her marginality (Mander, 1997). Cause and effect are here closely intertwined for the direct entry midwife because of her need to practise secretly with limited peer support and no formal organisation (DeVries & Barroso, 1997: 256).

Thus, the heterogeneity of the American midwife has been a threat to her survival not only historically, but also in the recent past. Recent conflicts have featured the near-suicidal competition between the direct entry midwife and the CNM. It may be that this competitive relationship is now being resolved. A stereotypically American characteristic, competition is advocated in many aspects of American life, including health care. This characteristic is explained in terms of the USA being an individual rights-based society in which competition is paramount and power is decentralised (Enthoven, 1994: 1422). The competitive nature of maternity care is aggravated by an overprovision of services in general and a physician oversupply in particular (Ham *et al.*, 1990; Ginzberg, 1998). This scenario is supported by Declercq's figures which show that the USA has 35 000 obstetricians and 4000 CNMs/midwives, whereas in the UK there are 3000 obstetricians and 35 000 midwives (Declercq, 1998: 459).

Against this background it may not be surprising that these two groups of midwives have been locked in long term and possibly ongoing competition. The CNM's viewpoint is more comprehensively documented and features anxiety about the safety of the direct entry midwife's practice and her lack of formal training. This poor relationship has been further hampered by the CNM's cosy dependence on her medical colleagues, even though medical support for the CNM is by no means universal (Bourgeault & Fynes, 1997: 1054). The near fatal outcome of the counterproductive competition within USA midwifery is widely recognised. It provides a stark example of a profession whose progress is impeded through internal divisions. As Declercq observes, the finite resources utilised by this internecine competition would have been better 'applied to the growth of American midwifery in general' (Declercq, 1994: 234).

Another aspect of competition which affected maternity care in the USA related to the problem of medical litigation, which has already been mentioned in the Canadian context. The relatively early and more urgent opting out of USA physicians from maternity care provided the CNM, who was sufficiently organised to do so, with an opportunity to take advantage of this 'gap in the market' or, in the terms of Abbott (1988), to 'occupy the vacant jurisdiction'. This, in competitive terms, admirable manoeuvre achieved 'dual closure' by occupying the vacancy left by the obstetrician at the same time as excluding the direct entry midwife from making progress (Bourgeault & Fynes,1997: 1060).

Because of her entrepreneurial orientation the CNM may be regarded as relatively independent in her practice and of high status. Whether this is actually the case depends on her relationship with both her medical 'back-up' and with her nursing colleagues in the LDR (labour and delivery room) (Mander, 1997). For the CNM who practises as part of a group alongside physicians, who provide her back-up, her status may be uncertain. This is because she is likely to be employed by the physicians, reducing her status to merely that of an employee, rather than a partner. For the CNM who is employed by a large charitable organisation, her status probably equates with that of a UK midwife working within an NHS trust, although the explicitly competitive nature of USA maternity care may make the CNM's employment less secure. The CNM must, inevitably, negotiate her role with the LDR nurses alongside whom she works and as one of whom her career may have begun. The different views about childbearing which led the CNM to leave the ranks of the LDR nurses provide fertile ground for conflict. This may affect the care of the individual woman as it is the LDR nurse, who works full time in the maternity unit, who decides when to contact the CNM who is on call (Mander, 1997).

It is apparent that the CNM's status is not entirely clear and may be described as marginal. In some ways this is similar to the way the direct entry midwife is described (DeVries & Barroso, 1997; Mander, 1997). The direct entry midwife's marginality is attributable largely to her, possibly formerly, illegal status. This may be moderated by the midwife's endeavours to establish good working relationships with local nursing and medical personnel who facilitate her practice for the benefit of her client. For the CNM and the direct entry midwife, the organisation of USA health care means that her autonomy, like her status, varies according to her working situation.

In the USA it is clear that the CNM was in a position to respond to the demands of the women's movement, while the direct entry midwife was still too weak and insufficiently organised to do so (Bourgeault & Fynes, 1997: 1060). Although the woman in the USA may have been in a strong position to exert her wishes regarding who provides maternity care through this powerful mass movement, the power of the individual woman is another matter. The limited choice of the American consumer of health care in general and of maternity care in particular is legendary. This lack of choice is apparent in the context of one highly contentious neonatal intervention, male circumcision, which is likely to comprise part of the 'insurance package' and, hence, be routine. Such a questionable arrangement has been termed 'insurance-led treatment' (Mander 1997: 1193). Other less gruesome examples of insurance companies taking decisions which would rightly be taken by the woman include the duration of her stay in the maternity unit post natally (Declercq, 1998: 852). This is a decision which should depend on the confidence as well as the health of the mother and baby. Insurers, however, take account only of severe illness if the discharge of the mother and baby to a relatively unsupportive home environment is to be delayed.

Although the discussion of the woman's choice in the USA has related to insurance schemes, it is necessary to recall that such schemes provide far from universal coverage (Ginzberg, 1998). This means that a large proportion is contributed by the client's or the patient's out-of-pocket expenses. The failure of the Clinton health system reforms, a cornerstone of which was at least a move towards universal health care coverage, has been explained thus:

> 'The public with adequate health insurance saw themselves as losers under a system of expanded coverage and that perception sufficed to kill the reform efforts.'

> (Ginzberg, 1998: 502)

The concept of equity is lacking at governmental policy level as well as in purely individual matters, such as the choice of the place of birth. For the insured woman care in labour is in a spacious room with a panoramic view over the bay. Her friend on Medicaid, however, may labour in a windowless room with space only for the woman's bed and the monitor (Mander, 1997: 1193). It is apparent that inequity features prominently on the American health care agenda, and that this notorious 'paradox of excesses and deprivation' (Enthoven, 1989) shows little sign of being resolved.

The American woman's experience of childbirth is determined by the method of payment. For the woman who is covered by private health insurance, her medical care, including the birth, is likely to be provided by 'her' physician. If her insurance permits or if local contracts are in place she may have access to a CNM group practice or one comprising physicians and CNMs; if the latter is the case, the woman will not know in advance whether her care will be by a CNM or a physician as on-call systems operate (Mander, 1997). With this level of uncertainty it may not be surprising that women sometimes use the yellow pages or the local women's network in order to locate a direct entry midwife. In this way at least continuity of carer will be assured.

The Netherlands

As already shown, the Dutch midwife seems to have been ideally positioned to ensure her survival in relation to, particularly, her medical colleagues. I now examine the factors which have put this midwife in such a strong position and those groups who may or may not have helped her. The role of the Dutch local authorities and the state have been crucial in supporting the midwife. First, this was by favouring her regulation rather than that of her medical colleagues. Second, the state ensured her continuing provision of home birth by legislating for the maternity home care assistant (MHCA) (van Teijlingen & van der Hulst, 1995: 182).

In the same way as medical practitioners have supported the continuation of the midwife in other countries, such as the UK, in order to achieve their own differing ends, the Dutch midwife has been assisted thus:

> '...without the protection of influential gynaecologists/obstetricians, it is likely that Dutch midwifery would look much like midwifery in other industrialised nations.'

> (DeVries & Barroso, 1997: 253)

That this source of support is likely to be withdrawn is mentioned by van Teij-lingen (1994: 109). Hingstman (1994) also suggests that competition has already become a feature of Dutch maternity care. In this unusual three way pattern of competition, it is the general practitioner who has been the loser. His share of the 'obstetric market' has traditionally been in the hands of the midwife (Hingstman, 1994: 84). It will remain to be seen whether the Dutch midwife is able to survive, not only without the support of her obstetrician colleagues, but in the face of the competition with which that support already appears to be being supplanted.

As mentioned above the system known as *primaat* means that the woman is encouraged by financial inducements to employ the services of a midwife, if there is one in practice in her locality. Although obviously favourable to the midwife, this system may be interpreted as limiting the woman's right to choose freely her childbirth attendant.

A choice which the Dutch woman is free to make relates to the place of birth (Jabaaij & Meijer, 1996). She is able to choose to be attended by a midwife either at home or in a polyclinic (a short stay maternity unit) with no financial sanctions. DeVries and Barroso (1997: 261) report the increasing popularity of this arrangement where there is '*alles bij de hand*' – meaning that everything, including facilities for medical intervention, is easily available. This changing picture is disconcerting for two reasons. First, the traditional power base of the Dutch midwife, the home birth, appears to be being undermined. Second, the culture which convinces the Dutch woman of the likely successful functioning of her body in labour, mentioned earlier, is also undergoing a change. The Dutch midwife is responding actively to these perceived threats by developing a practice which is more scientific without becoming more technological. An example relating to the woman's choice of place of birth is given by DeVries and Barroso (1997) to illustrate the high status of the Dutch midwife. In the light of the threatening changes mentioned above, these authors describe the midwife's response to correct the situation. It may involve challenging the woman to explain her reasons for seeking to give birth in a polyclinic. Extraordinarily, this challenge bears some comparison with the interrogation which women in some countries, such as the UK, often face when seeking a home birth.

The relatively high status of the Dutch midwife compared with her UK or north American counterpart may be due to a number of characteristics. These include, first, the high barriers to entry into the profession which she needs to overcome (Tasharroffi, 1993). Second, the Dutch midwife's entrepreneurial status may serve to elevate her to the social standing of those with whom she is in competition (Mander, 1995: 1025). Third, the level of commitment required to make a living may further elevate her status above that of a midwife who is an employee. Fourth, the existence of the MHCA as an assistant elevates the mid-wife's occupational status (Mander, 1995).

The existence of the MHCA assisting the Dutch midwife's relatively high status brings to mind the possibility of a hierarchy operating. Such a scenario would feature the low status tasks being undertaken by an attendant who remains with the woman while the higher status tasks are assumed by another attendant who appears at the appropriate point in the pregnancy, birth or post natal period. An example of the help which would be given by the MHCA is advising about the resumption of sexual relations post natally (van Teijlingen & McCaffery, 1987). The authors maintain that it would not be appropriate for the midwife to provide this advice due to the midwife's social distance from the mother. Thus, concern is aroused that the ability of the Dutch midwife to be 'with woman' may actually be hampered by her high status. This means that the gaps in her midwifery care are plugged by a less qualified and more easily accessible attendant. These concerns are further aggravated by the account of the midwife's intermittent attendance when a woman labours at home (Jabaaij & Meijer, 1996). Again, the picture emerges of a discontinuous form of care, with the midwife 'dropping in' during the labour. The similarities between this pattern of intrapartum care and that offered by the labour delivery room nurse and the physician in the USA are difficult to ignore.

It appears that the Dutch system of maternity care has many aspects which are admirable in their ability to ensure that the woman is able to make crucial choices. Even this system, however, is not without its areas of weakness in the form of potential threats and changes which have already begun to happen.

Discussion

What emerges from this examination of health care systems in general and three systems of maternity care in particular is their similarities and their differences. Although the name, midwife, is widely used, the actual function and other characteristics of that person vary considerably. Other similarities which have emerged relate to the widespread search for efficiency in health care, which is resulting in a focus on limiting or reducing costs. This search is also associated with what has been termed an 'epidemic' of reforms to health care systems.

The comparisons which I have been able to draw in this chapter should be considered in the context of general data on the health care systems involved. In view of the importance which governments have been shown to attach to the reduction of health care costs, the relative expenditure deserves attention. The American health care bill is more than twice that in the UK (per capita UK = $1365, US = $3708; proportion of GDP UK = 6.9%, US = 14.2%). In spite of this, mortality rates in the USA are consistently higher than in the UK (Declercq, 1998: 835).

More general comparisons of the maternity care systems in Canada, the USA and UK are drawn by Simkin and Ancheta (2000: 6–7). These authors list:

- Primary maternity caregivers
- Autonomy/independence of caregiver
- Childbearing woman's input into decision-making

- Continuity of caregiver
- Influence of scientific evidence on practice
- Influence of malpractice litigation.

Clearly these comparisons are considered to be significant. Unfortunately, apart from the numerical data, the comparisons which are given are too superficial to inform this hugely complex area.

The differences between the systems of maternity care appear to be attributable, as Jordan (1978: 73) observes, to this aspect of life being part of a larger cultural system and part of an even larger ideology. The conclusion that these systems and ideologies are being influenced to some extent by medicalisation is difficult to avoid. In the examples which I have discussed this process appears to be at different stages and there may actually be a backlash in some areas.

The material which I have examined in this chapter has shown the likely influence of the health care system on maternity care. This in turn affects the variety of ways in which the midwife is able to provide supportive care for the childbearing woman. In the next chapter the focus is on that support, before moving on in Chapter 4 to the support which the midwife has been shown to provide. This chapter's material on systems of health care is used as the context for the examination in Chapter 5 of the research on support in labour and in Chapter 6 of the operationalisation of that research.

Chapter 3
The provision of support during childbearing

In the first two chapters of this book I considered the nature of social support and then the extent to which it may be facilitated in the context of certain health care systems, with particular reference to maternity care. It is now necessary to examine the links between these discrete phenomena. In this chapter I first examine the need for support, in the form of the factors associated with negative stress during the childbearing cycle. This is followed by the role and provision of support at different points and by different personnel during a woman's childbearing experience. I begin, though, with a relatively wide-ranging examination of childbearing stress before focusing on the details of when and who.

Stress in childbearing

I have made brief reference in Chapter 1 to the role of negative stress in relation to each individual's need for support. It may be helpful to examine separately stress in childbearing in view of its unique features and implications. Chapters 5 and 6 focus more precisely on labour, so here I mention only briefly intrapartum events which may be stressful.

Stress in pregnancy

The prevalence of stress-related problems in pregnancy is undergoing marked change. This is due in no small part to the introduction of programmes of pre-natal screening and other tests during pregnancy. These programmes may be regarded as reassuring. In this way they may have actually reduced some of the negative stressors and anxieties to which the pregnant woman is vulnerable. On the other hand, there may be an element of iatrogenesis, as some of these stressors may have been supplanted by others which are engendered specifically by the testing regime itself (Scott & Niven, 1996).

As well as the obvious immediate and long term hazards for the woman's health, negative stress in pregnancy carries serious risks for the welfare of the baby. The fetal implications have been shown to operate through the trans-placental transfer of stress-related hormones, such as the catecholamines. These hormones are likely to affect the fetus in two ways. First, they reduce placental perfusion and, hence, fetal oxygenation. Second, they also increase the contractility of the uterine musculature, the myometrium. In this way, stressful life events have been shown to be associated with intrauterine growth retardation, premature labour and birth. For these reasons the woman who suffers excessive negative stress may give birth to a baby of low birth weight (LBW – less than 2.5 kilos).

Newton (1988) emphasises the vulnerability of certain groups of women to life's stressors. This vulnerability is likely to be exacerbated if the woman has relatively limited access to coping resources. These groups include women who are aged less than 20 years at three months' gestation, women who are unsupported by a stable relationship and those whose employment status categorises them as being in socio-economic class four or five. There are other important psychosocial factors, which are likely to act as stressors and which are also associated with LBW. These factors may not operate independently of those mentioned already, as they may be used as coping strategies. They include cigarette smoking and alcohol and other substance abuse. The complexity of the relationship between these various stressors became apparent in the research by Newton and Hunt (1984) which indicated a positive correlation between smoking and poor clinic attendance and low birth weight.

Whether the effects of stress are direct or are mediated through the woman's perceptions is not entirely clear. Scott and Niven (1996) suggest a cognitive appraisal framework involving the woman's perception of the stressfulness of an event or experience. Recent transcultural research in the USA, however, suggests a direct link between sociocultural context and birth weight (Rini *et al.*, 1999). Regardless of the mechanism, though, the link between stress and low birth weight appears to be well-established through observational studies. In this way the ground was prepared for important intervention studies which aimed to assess the effects of support on both stress and birth weight (see later in this chapter).

Stress in labour

As I mentioned in the introduction to this section I give little attention here to stress in labour, partly because Chapters 5 and 6 focus intensively on the events of labour, and partly because the research and other literature on labour as being a stressful experience is seriously limited. This neglect of any association between stress and labour is in spite of labour pain having been shown to be at least as intense as the pain of cancer (Melzack & Wall, 1991: 43).

The exceptions to this observation of neglect are interesting. Stress in labour is usually mentioned briefly and generally in textbooks on care in childbirth (Piotrowski, 1997: 360; Cassidy, 1999: 400). The use of the term stress in these publications is so general as to be meaningless, as it reflects little more than unfocused anxiety. Of greater value is the research by Annie and Groer (1991), which assessed stress during childbirth by using immunological measurements. The findings, however, have limited input into the mother's care.

The research and other material which is widely used to advocate support in labour does tend to draw on the concept of stress, but not the name. Examples are found in the research reports by Sosa and colleagues (1980: 600) and by Klaus and colleagues (1986: 587). In hypothesising why support in labour may be effective, these researchers discuss the role of catecholamines, but fail to mention their crucial role in the stress response. Further, the Dublin regime discusses 'panic' and the possibility of the labouring woman's 'total disintegration' (O'Driscoll *et al.*, 1993: 93) without mentioning the possibility of this experience being negatively stressful.

The reasons for the limited attention given to labour as a stressful experience are not clear. This neglect may be attributable to the relatively short term or acute nature of labour; but stress is not ordinarily defined in terms of being time limited. Another possible explanation is that labour features both positive and negative aspects whereas stress currently tends to be viewed only negatively, which again is not an accurate representation of this phenomenon.

Stress in the post natal period

The experience of the woman in the post natal period has recently been attracting the research attention which it has long deserved. As well as pathophysiological conditions, the woman's psychosocial state is also the focus of interest. A largely qualitative study of social support in the post natal period was undertaken using feminist research methodology (Podkolinski, 1998). While preparing for this study the researcher examined the increase in negative stressors which women are likely to encounter at the time of adjustment to motherhood. Particularly significant now, in view of women's more frenetic lifestyle, is the demise of the 'lying-in' period. This period of 'confinement', when the woman traditionally allows herself to rest and be pampered, facilitates her 'babying' her baby. Podkolinski is able to draw an all too clear distinction between the restful, restorative lying-in period and the post natal stay in hospital. She argues that, in spite of the best efforts of the staff, the post natal ward is unlikely to offer a sufficiently stress-free environment to permit recuperation and to initiate adjustment to new motherhood.

The cultural underpinning of the post natal period is crucial to our understanding and provision of care at this time (Cheung, 1997). It may be argued that due to the absence of ritual the stress of the transition to motherhood is unmitigated. This argument is less than convincing because the loss of ritual may mean no more than one set of rituals being replaced by another set. These include the carefully stage-managed introduction of the older child to the new baby. Another example is the proud 'reunion' for those who attended childbirth education sessions. It may be that the woman's fraught first experience of leaving her baby in the care of another person, perhaps when she returns to her paid employment, is another. The new rituals or rites of passage, however, may be perceived as less effective than the old ones, which would include community activities such as the baptism. There may still be benefit, though, in their role of relieving the individual of the burden of having to make decisions at stressful times, such as during the transition to motherhood.

Post natal stress was assessed indirectly by a quantitative study, which measured women's satisfaction with the extent to which they had resumed their usual functional status post natally (McVeigh, 1997). A convenience sample of two hundred Australian women completed the Inventory of Functional Status After Childbirth (IFSAC) (Fawcett *et al.*, 1988). McVeigh shows clearly the women's disappointingly slow return to their normal functioning on a range of criteria, including household, social, childcare, selfcare, and occupational activities. While not explicitly stating the stressful nature of such a slow recovery, this researcher indicates that better support would have assisted the woman's recuperation. The dissatisfaction that these women encountered was related particularly to their reduced feelings of well-being and to their interrupted patterns of sleep.

This relative deterioration in the woman's function and the associated feelings also manifested themselves in a study in England (Herbert, 1994). A prospective, longitudinal exploratory study involved 24 first time mothers, each of whom completed two questionnaires, a diary and four semistructured interviews. This researcher, like McVeigh, omits to mention stress, referring to each mother's profound tiredness, social isolation and anxiety about the baby's well-being. Again, like McVeigh, Herbert suggests that social support would have remedied the less than satisfactory situations in which these women found themselves.

The effects of support in childbearing

While preparing for her major study on social support in childbearing, Oakley (1988) questioned whether social support is good for the health of mothers and babies. She used ante natal care as an example of the medical model in operation in having as one of its major aims the prevention of the birth of LBW babies. Using this model the link has been established in true Cartesian style between birth weight and social factors. Inevitably, Oakley sought to build on research mentioned earlier in this chapter which links higher rates of LBW with lower socio-economic class. Oakley and colleagues' research attempted to identify the means whereby social factors influence the development and the birth weight of the baby (Oakley *et al.*, 1990). These researchers were also seeking to assess the extent to which supportive interventions might be effective in ameliorating this influence.

Oakley drew on the work of Newton and Hunt (1984) which indicated a link between lower socio-economic class and more and more severe life events. On this basis she hypothesised that social support may operate in one or more of a number of ways.

(1) It may have a direct benefit on health
(2) Social support may indirectly serve to lessen the harm which is caused by stress
(3) It may decrease the risk of exposure to stress
(4) It may facilitate recovery from stressful conditions such as illness.

Her analysis of observation and intervention studies undertaken during the previous decade showed consistently beneficial effects of support on psychosocial outcomes. This conclusion, however, was seriously impeded by the studies' lack of methodological rigour. All too frequently the researchers' enthusiasm had caused them to ignore certain confounding factors, including the 'Hawthorne effect' that is the participants' perceived benefit due to involvement in a research project and the anticipation of a gentle birth. Similarly, the previous researchers' need to establish the link between support and improved outcomes prevented them from considering the nature of the *process* which led to those outcomes.

Drawing on this general research background, Oakley and colleagues (1990) undertook a randomised controlled trial (RCT) to study the effects of social support on birth weight. The hypothesis stated that social support would increase the birth weight of the babies by an average of 150 g. Women with a history of giving birth to LBW babies were recruited from four maternity units. As well as childbearing criteria, a woman could only be recruited into the study if she was able to speak English fluently. The process of randomisation resulted in an intervention group of 255 women designated to receive social support in addition to routine care. The control group comprised 254 women who were allocated to receive only routine care.

The social support package offered to the intervention group comprised a minimum of three home visits by the research midwife employed at the maternity unit which the woman attended. Additionally there were two brief contacts and a 24 hour on-call help-line. The women were encouraged to discuss any pregnancy-related issues which were of concern to them. The midwife was permitted to give advice or information only on specific topics and only when explicitly asked to do so. The midwife did not provide clinical midwifery care but was able to make referrals. The pregnancy outcomes were measured by reference to the woman's medical notes and by a postal questionnaire at six weeks after the birth.

The data showed that the two groups were comparable in terms of the women's personal characteristics. The experiment group of women were happy with their support, reporting that the midwife listened and that this was considered helpful. The women in the control group were admitted to hospital significantly more frequently than those in the experiment group. The babies born to the intervention group were of higher birth weight and these mothers and babies were healthier post natally. The women in the control group also appreciated their involvement in the study, which may have affected the results by reducing the difference between the two groups.

The finding that the supported women's babies were on average only 38 g larger than the control group's babies meant that the hypothesis failed to be supported. The fact that the women in the intervention group enjoyed better health throughout their childbearing experience led Oakley and colleagues to question whether this was a direct effect or whether it was mediated by greater confidence and happiness. Clearly these researchers were unable to increase babies' birth weight to the hypothesised level. In spite of this they felt able to conclude that reduction in the incidence of LBW is amenable to action other than just strictly health care interventions. Thus, Oakley and colleagues consider that social interventions are also effective.

A scheme of providing additional social support to pregnant women in Manchester who were at increased risk of giving birth to a LBW baby produced similar findings (Spencer *et al.*, 1989). This study was also an RCT but, unlike Oakley's, the support was provided by a lay person, known as a family worker. No significant difference in the birth weight of the babies was observed between the intervention group and the control group.

The possibility of using the findings of Oakley and colleagues' study in other cultures is uncertain, as reflected in Langer and colleagues' (1996) RCT involving 2235 women at high risk of giving birth to LBW babies in four Latin American institutions. The trial aimed to evaluate a psychosocial support intervention during pregnancy which sought to improve perinatal health and the woman's psychosocial circumstances. The intervention comprised four to six home visits, during which emotional support, counselling and strengthening of the woman's social network were offered. Data were collected at 36 weeks of pregnancy, early in the post natal period and at 40 days after the birth. These researchers found no significant differences between the two groups' perceptions of social support and satisfaction with the childbearing experience, or with the maternal and neonatal care. Langer and colleagues concluded that something more than psychosocial interventions during pregnancy is required to resolve maternal-child health problems in developing countries.

That the effectiveness of support is in some way linked to the local level of industrialisation is supported by a Northern Californian study involving 319 African-American women (Norbeck *et al.*, 1996). This environment clearly has more in common with that of Oakley and colleagues' research than that by Langer and colleagues. Using focus groups in mid-pregnancy, Norbeck and colleagues identified women who lacked support either from their mother or from a male partner. The intervention aimed to provide the support ordinarily offered by these significant others; this comprised four face-to-face sessions as well as intervening telephone contacts. The rate of LBW was found by scrutiny of documents to be 9.1% in the intervention group compared with 22.4% in the control group. On the grounds of this significant reduction in the LBW rate ($p < 0.05$), Norbeck and colleagues conclude that support is effective in reducing the incidence of this major problem among this relatively prosperous population.

Support in pregnancy

The important work which has been undertaken by researchers such as Oakley and colleagues (1990) has examined the effect of support on the entire childbearing experience. Other work has focused more precisely on specific periods during that experience, such as pregnancy.

In her account of psychosocial support in pregnancy, Wheatley (1998: 50) draws on research by Schumaker and Brownell (1984) to explain its effectiveness. These researchers identified the mutual or interactional components which determine the benefit or damage associated with support. Examples of these components include, first, the person–environment fit which refers to the acceptability and availability of support to the recipient. Second, the perception of the balance of the transaction may affect the support's effectiveness, such as through perceptions of inadequate help being offered. Third is the nature of the support and its appropriateness, for example the misfit of psychological support being offered when more instrumental support is sought. Fourth, the temporal nature of the support may determine its effectiveness, such as short term intensive support having the potential to create long term dependency.

Wheatley considers that when each of these components suits both the supporter and the supported, the likely outcome is a positive influence on the individual's emotional well-being. Thus, in pregnancy such support would engender confidence in the woman that she is adequately prepared for her childbearing experience, whatever form it assumes. In this way anxiety and depression are likely to be reduced. If the support is not appropriate to the pregnant woman in terms of one or more of the four components, the beneficial effects may be reversed. The result is likely to be harm to the woman's emotional health with the possibility of depression both during pregnancy and post natally.

Research on the effects of support by a wide range of caregivers during 'at-risk pregnancy' was subjected to systematic review by Hodnett (2000a). She identified 14 trials employing suitably rigorous research methods and involving over 11 000 women. A wide range of outcomes were found to have been measured. These included 'medical' outcomes, such as preterm birth, pregnancy outcome, LBW, interventions in labour and perinatal mortality. Hodnett found that 'medical' outcomes were not changed by social support. Immediate psychosocial outcomes, though, such as anxiety, dissatisfaction and help-seeking behaviours, were more likely to be improved.

Hodnett hypothesises several reasons for these indeterminate findings. First, the social support provided may be inadequate to overcome the severe long term deprivation of the 'at risk' women recruited into the studies. Alternatively, the criteria for inclusion into the studies may not have been sufficiently sensitive to identify women who were actually at high risk, resulting in the non-significant findings. Although Hodnett refers to the 'effects of a lifetime of poverty and disadvantage', this systematic review does not consider the potential for longer term benefits of social support.

Support in the post natal period

The role of the midwife and the supportive nature of midwifery care is examined in Chapter 4. Here the research on specific support which may be given by a range of carers is addressed.

A qualitative study of post natal support, mentioned in the earlier section on post natal stress (Podkolinski, 1998) examined the post natal experiences of ten women. Each woman lived with a male partner, who with the baby's grandmother provided most of the support. The woman experienced intensive support from these sources for a period ranging from six to seventeen days. The women preferred their support to be by someone who was at least their age and also a mother. This researcher identified that practical support, in the form of helping with housework, is as important as emotional support. The partner's support was found to vary in the extent to which it met the woman's expectations. Podkolinski gives examples of partners who were thought to expect too much of the new mother. This research shows the crucial nature of the support offered by women in the post natal period to the new mother – 'It did not matter whether they were relatives, friends or professionals' (Podkolinski, 1998: 221). For each of the new mothers, her ability to locate effective and timely support was clearly a source of some surprise to her.

A recent study in Scotland sought to assess the relative benefits of certain frequently used supportive interventions (Reid, 1997). This study aimed to correct the lack of evidence relating to the effectiveness of post natal support groups as well as assessing the efficiency of interventions at this time. The sample comprised 1004 women, who were recruited in two areas.

This RCT investigated the effects of group support, an information pack and a combination of the two as compared with a control group who received neither. The group support involved a facilitator/researcher who encouraged the women to discuss psychological issues and practical topics, such as baby care. Although the discussion was facilitated by a researcher, the agenda was decided by the women. The information pack comprised illustrated booklets which encouraged the woman to accept the difficulties which a new mother is likely to encounter. Data collection was by three sets of questionnaires which sought information on a range of topics, including physical health, post natal depression, costs of group attendance and use of health services. The economic evaluation sought as far as possible to adopt a user perspective, such as the opportunity costs of attending a post natal support group.

The response rate was generally good, ranging from 88% to 71%. The women who participated tended to be older and of higher socio-economic class, although not significantly. As has been found in other forms of group activity, women of higher socio-economic class were more likely to attend the group support sessions. When those women who chose not to attend were asked why, they stated that the sessions were not convenient in terms of time and/or venue. Reid and her colleagues (1999) found no significant differences in terms of health outcomes and health service usage among the four groups of women. The health data indicate that the costs of providing support groups, which may not be well attended by those for whom they are intended, may not be justified.

The provision of support

In her study of the post natal experiences of 24 first time mothers, Herbert (1994) found that support was most likely to be found with the baby's grandmother, friends and other new mothers. The grandmother was seen as variably supportive. While her help with household chores was universally welcomed, Herbert found that her involvement tended to be viewed with concern in case it escalated into interference. Visiting by friends was not universally welcome because of the woman's inability to control how long visitors stayed. The length of visits was found to be likely to aggravate the woman's overwhelming complaint of tiredness. Each of the new mothers reported that her circle of friends changed over the first three months of the baby's life. She found that she was able to find more appropriate support, including reassurance of normality, from other mothers rather than her previous friends.

Although in Herbert's study the woman's partner did not feature as particularly significant in the provision of post natal support, McVeigh (1997) found that the partner's support did matter. As other researchers had identified previously, McVeigh revealed a vicious cycle of interrupted sleep pattern, tiredness, dissatisfaction with well-being, poor support and social isolation. She argues that women should be taught to 'actively enlist' appropriate support in advance of it being needed (McVeigh, 1997: 177). McVeigh implies that the woman's high expectation for her own independent performance in other aspects of her life is applied to motherhood, resulting in a downward spiral of diminishing well-being.

The supportive role of the partner as well as the grandmother also emerged as crucial in the observational study by Podkolinski (1998). For the woman whose partner did not match up to her expectations, the emotional support of other experienced women was greatly valued. This applied particularly to those women who through relatively insignificant actions, such as a bed bath, were made to feel 'special'. In the same way as certain supportive actions made the woman feel good, other well intended actions could have the reverse effect. In these situations intended support could be perceived as interference, which would prevent the woman from seeking help in future. Just as Herbert found, Podkolinski's sample regarded visitors as a mixed blessing. The extent of the need for support was unexpectedly high for both the woman and her partner, although there were variations in the relative proportions of practical and emotional help which each of the couple needed. Podkolinski, like McVeigh, identified the common and largely self-generated expectation that the woman would be able to cope alone with the transition to motherhood. This is comparable to the way she is accustomed to coping with challenging experiences in her working life. Unfortunately these high expectations of her own performance meant that any offers of help soon ceased to be forthcoming.

Debriefing

An intervention to reduce psychological morbidity has been recommended following a number of potentially disturbing experiences, including childbirth. This intervention has become known, perhaps inappropriately according to Alexander (1998), as 'debriefing'.

Originally introduced to facilitate the recovery of survivors of mass disasters, such as the sinking of the ship *Herald of Free Enterprise*, it has become a routine intervention for emergency personnel and the victims of trauma such as road traffic accidents or assaults (Wessely *et al.*, 2000). The need for debriefing post natally has been suggested in view of the potential for psychological disturbance following an unexpectedly traumatic birth experience (Crompton, 1996). This intervention has also been suggested for more general use with new mothers; in this context debriefing may in itself constitute support, or it may be a method of identifying a woman's support needs (Alexander, 1998: 122).

While Alexander questions both the clarity of terminology and the appropriateness of debriefing, its highly structured nature may also impede its widespread use post natally. Based on the work of Dyregrov (1989), Curtis (1995) suggests that this structure comprises eight stages:

(1) Identification
(2) Labelling
(3) Articulation
(4) Expression
(5) Externalisation
(6) Ventilation
(7) Validation
(8) Acceptance.

Essentially, debriefing seeks to normalise the affected person's emotional response in an attempt to view it as a healthy reaction to a traumatic event. Alexander reviewed the research on the effectiveness of debriefing in childbearing situations. She found no evidence to suggest that debriefing is effective in reducing psychological morbidity. On the basis of examining literature relating to both civilian and military debriefing, the systematic review by Wessely and colleagues (2000) drew very similar conclusions. Of particular concern is these researchers' comment after their conclusion of unproven effectiveness; bearing in mind the vulnerability of the client group, they sound an appropriately warning note to the effect that:

'The possibility of adverse effects must be remembered.'

(Wessely *et al.*, 2000: 15)

Support after perinatal bereavement

The woman who has lost a baby through death or in another way has particular support needs. These needs are partly attributable to the likelihood of the development of some form of pathological grief.

The effects of supportive care on the resolution of grief following perinatal death were the subject of an RCT by Forrest and colleagues (1982). Fifty mothers of babies who had died perinatally were recruited; half of the mothers received 'ideal' supported care, while the 'contrast' group received care of the usual uncertain standard. The supported group were encouraged to see, hold and name their dead baby. Photographs were taken of the baby. The mother chose, whenever possible, where she was cared for and her transfer home was unhurried. Bereavement counselling was offered to both parents within two days of their loss.

The counselled mothers recovered from their grief more quickly than the contrast group. Forrest and colleagues found, however, that by the fourteen month assessment there was no significant difference between the two groups. These findings are largely reassuring, though it may be that the intervention served only to 'hurry' the grief of the supported group. It is necessary to question, apart from the pain being longer lasting, whether marginally longer grief necessarily indicates less effective grief. The lack of detail of the nature of the support and the high attrition rate from the supported group also give rise to concern.

Although the family has been shown (above) to be important in providing support post natally, their limited ability to provide suitable support for the bereaved mother has emerged in a number of studies. The 22 bereaved mothers in Alice Lovell's sample found that their friends and family had other preoccupations which limited the support they could make available (Lovell, 1983). Disconcertingly, Lovell found that the bereaved grandmother was the least able to comfort the mother (p. 326), perhaps due to her own grief over the loss of her grandchild.

Rajan and Oakley (1993) in the course of the major study mentioned earlier in the section 'The effects of support in childbearing' (Oakley *et al.*, 1990) identified similarly unsupportive reactions. Eighty-four previously bereaved mothers were included in this large and authoritative sample. These researchers found that the male partner experienced loss in his own way and was unlikely to share the mother's need to articulate her loss or to express it in other ways. The need for the grieving mother to support her partner and others close to her tended to result in her delaying her own grieving. They found that the woman tended to put everyone's needs before her own. Thus Rajan and Oakley showed the lack of support for the mother, whose need is likely to be greatest, while she is providing support for those near to her. People whom the mother had previously regarded as friends were found to be unable to cope with facing her when she had been bereaved. As a result contact was avoided to the extent of literally crossing the road to avoid having to speak.

Thus, the grieving mothers interviewed by Lovell (1983) found that 'community support' is far less caring and comforting than the name may imply and this finding is fully endorsed by Rajan and Oakley's more recent data. Lovell's findings led her to the conclusion that the grieving mother might have been better supported if she had remained longer in the maternity unit.

A large retrospective study of stillbirth in Sweden (Rådestad *et al.*, 1996) included items in the questionnaire on the support available. Of a range of health care and other personnel in a position to offer support, the social worker was most frequently mentioned as helpful (41% of women, $n = 129$). A large majority of the women (64%, $n = 203$) were either 'quite' or 'entirely' satisfied with their support. In view of this finding, it is surprising that 21% of the women ($n = 67$) stated that they had been able to locate 'no support at all'.

Clearly support is much appreciated by the bereaved mother and its absence is a source of regret. The evidence of its effectiveness in the prevention of pathological grief, though, is lacking. On the basis of their systematic review, Chambers and Chan (2000: 5) conclude that:

> 'No information is available from randomised trials to indicate whether there is or is not a benefit from providing specific psychological support or counselling after perinatal death.'

Post natal depression

The condition which has become known as post natal depression is perplexing to all involved. Those who provide care continue to debate its cause. The timing and existence of this psychiatric illness have been questioned (Green, 1998). There is uncertainty about its incidence, which is due to the difficulty of the depressed new mother either not realising that she has a problem, not realising that her problem is amenable to help or not being able to seek help. Elliott (1989) showed clearly the serious implications of post natal depression. These include long term effects on the mother's health and well-being, effects on the child's behaviour and effects on the woman's relationships.

Following her major study on social support in childbearing, Oakley (1992b) drew attention to post natal depression. She found that inadequate social support, that is perceived as such by the woman herself, may lower her emotional well-being. Post natal depression may follow, which may last until the baby is at least one year old. As well as lack of support being a possible cause of post natal depression, support has been investigated as a therapeutic intervention to either prevent or treat it. Following their systematic review, Ray and Hodnett (2000) report that home-based social support for disadvantaged mothers and babies post natally has been found to reduce the mothers' feelings of unhappiness.

Support by the health visitor in the form of counselling to treat post natal depression was investigated in an RCT by Holden and colleagues (1989). The women's depression was diagnosed by screening when the baby was six weeks old. The Edinburgh Post Natal Depression Scale was used. The woman's response to eight weekly counselling sessions by a specially trained health visitor was assessed blind by a psychiatric interview at 13 weeks. Attrition was high, comprising five women who declined to participate and five women who did not complete the trial. The full recovery rate was 69% ($n = 18$ out of 26) in the counselling group, compared with 38% ($n = 9$ out of 24) in the control group. On the basis of these findings the researchers conclude that counselling support by a health visitor is effective in the treatment of post natal depression.

Appleby and colleagues (1997) compared counselling support with the administration of antidepressant medication (fluoxetine) in the treatment of post natal depression. This RCT was double blind for the medication administration. As in Holden and colleagues' study, Appleby and colleagues found a high attrition rate of 30% (n = 26 out of 87). The researchers found that all four treatment groups improved significantly, although the medication group's improvement was significantly better than the placebo group. The improvement was significantly better among the women who had six counselling sessions, compared with those who had only one session. The difference between the effects of the medication and the counselling was not significant. This finding leads the researchers to suggest that the woman should be able to choose either the medication or counselling support for the treatment of her post natal depression.

Breast feeding support

While support has been demonstrated to contribute to the woman's decision about *whether* to initiate breast feeding her baby (Thomson, 1989), it may be even more important in facilitating the *continuation* of breast feeding. An authoritative survey in England and Wales (Audit Commission, 1997) showed that 68% of women breast feed their babies at some time. The rapid discontinuation of breast feeding, however, is shown in the finding that only 30% were still doing so at three months. This duration needs to be viewed in the context of four to six months being generally recommended as the minimum age for a baby to be weaned from the breast in order to gain full immunological benefit (Howie, 1985).

The early work by Houston (1981) clearly showed the value of structured social support as an intervention which facilitates continuing breast feeding. Houston recruited the intervention group (n = 28) when the baby was three days old. Each woman was visited fortnightly by appointment until she discontinued breast feeding. During these visits the woman was encouraged to talk about feeding her baby and any problems which were developing. The control group (n = 52) was recruited retrospectively and was interviewed when the baby was 24 weeks old to ascertain whether breast feeding was continuing and, if not, why not.

Houston found that 100% of the supported women continued to feed beyond 12 weeks. By 24 weeks over 80% were still breast feeding, whereas the continuation rate for the controls was only 60%. Houston's additional observation of the increased likelihood of women of lower socio-economic class to discontinue breast feeding earlier is supported by more recent studies (ONS, 1997). Because of this finding, research focusing on social support has been undertaken in the hope of remedying the problem.

An exploratory study of breast feeding among women with a low income was completed by Whelan and Lupton (1998). These researchers identified the importance of the woman's expectations, especially whether they were realistic or not and whether influenced by childbirth education. A supportive social environment, including culture as well as family and friends, also proved important in breast feeding continuation. The support of other family members, particularly the grandmother, and friends was more valued than that of the partner. Whelan and Lupton found that the fathers in their study, with one exception, were not opposed to breast feeding. It was assumed that women with partners who were opposed would not even have attempted to breast feed and would have been ineligible. Each of the breast feeding women told the researchers of the supportive day-to-day help which her mother provided and also her mother-in-law, though to a lesser extent. It was found that experienced mothers were perceived as more supportive. Non-experienced mothers were not perceived as useful. The same observation also applied to friends with experience of breast feeding. Whelan and Lupton (1998: 97) found that the partner took a 'back seat' as far as breast feeding was concerned, which may be comparable with the observation of fathers 'postponing' their relationship with their offspring for the duration of breast feeding (Gamble & Morse, 1993).

The value of identifying one person who was supportive emerged as crucial in the study by Whelan and Lupton. That this person should be a woman was also clearly apparent. On the basis of these findings, the researchers make certain recommendations for the campaign to improve breast feeding rates among women of lower socio-economic class. They recommend that one individual support person, such as the woman's mother or, failing that, the partner, should be identified during pregnancy. The woman should aim to depend on this person for support after the birth. This person should then be fully involved in decision-making about infant feeding and in the woman's childbirth education.

Unlike Whelan and Lupton's observation, an intervention study was undertaken involving low income women in a North American city (Kistin *et al.*, 1994). This study examined the effect of support from trained peer counsellors on breast feeding initiation, duration and exclusivity. The counsellors provided information about health care issues including selfcare during breast feeding. The study compared breast feeding behaviour of women who planned to breast feed and received support from counsellors ($n = 59$) with women who requested counsellors but, due to inadequate numbers of trained counsellors, did not have access to one ($n = 43$). Women in the supported group had significantly greater (p < 0.05) breast feeding initiation (93% compared with 70%), exclusivity (77% compared with 40%), and duration (mean of 15 weeks compared with a mean of 8 weeks) than women in the unsupported group. The findings suggest that peer counsellors who are well-trained and provide on going support can have a positive effect on breast feeding behaviour among low-income urban women who intend to breast feed.

Research in developed countries has, at the time of writing, been focused on establishing the benefits of social support to the breast feeding woman, especially among women of lower socio-economic class. The Baby Friendly Initiative, however, has been introduced world wide (WHO/UNICEF, 1989). The introduction of this initiative in the UK may not always have been welcomed, and may occasionally have been viewed with 'indifference or hostility' (Palmer & Kemp, 1994: 14). It may be that the feelings of threat to which these authors refer are associated with the uncertainty described by Smale (1998). The largely fragmented nature of maternity care in the UK may prevent health care providers from considering the larger picture and the longer term effects of their advice. Thus Smale describes the dilemma facing some maternity unit staff in terms of 'woman or breast feeding?'. The short term difficulties which the woman initiating breast feeding may encounter are likely to become magnified to assume disproportionate importance in relation to the long term benefits. Hence 'short termism' may reduce the support which staff feel able to offer at what may be a challenging time for all involved, leading to unnecessarily high rates of discontinuation of breast feeding.

Informal carers

So far in this chapter I have examined the ways in which supportive care may be provided during the childbearing cycle by a range of professional carers. The role of informal carers also deserves attention, though this aspect of support may be less amenable to action by the maternity services. In this section I build on the literature on support by non-midwifery personnel, by focusing on certain informal carers whose input has been shown to be important.

First, though, it is necessary to examine and consider the implications of a published study which is likely to have considerable relevance. Webster and colleagues (2000) in Brisbane, Australia, undertook a large quantitative study which sought to assess the level of support provided by family and friends during pregnancy and to relate this support to post natal outcomes such as depression (PND). The researchers collected data from 2127 pregnant women attending the ante natal clinic and post natally from a sub sample of 600 women with risk factors for PND and 300 with none. The instruments comprised the Maternity Social Support Scale (MSSS) in pregnancy and the Edinburgh Post Natal Depression Scale. The MSSS was specially devised for this study and consisted of a Likert-type scale. It sought information on six topic areas:

(1)   Friends' support
(2)   Family support
(3)   Partner's help
(4)   Partner conflict
(5)   Control by partner
(6)   Partner's affection.

The pretesting of the MSSS was limited, only being reviewed for completeness by professionals and for acceptability by pregnant women. That the MSSS was acceptable to women, though, is reflected in the high response rate of 86.4%.

These researchers obtained information about the woman's perception of her situation and, more importantly, managed to open up the notoriously difficult area of domestic violence (Bewley, 1997). The researchers recognise the challenge which discussion of this area presents, especially in the context of a busy ante natal clinic. That the staff continued to use the MSSS after the completion of the research is a reflection of the value they attached to this instrument. The data showed that women who were less well supported experienced significantly poorer health during pregnancy ($p < 0.006$) and post natally ($p < 0.001$), as well as 'booking' significantly later ($p = 0.000$) for ante natal care and seeking medical advice significantly more frequently ($p = 0.004$). Webster and colleagues found that obstetric outcomes, such as mode of delivery or birth weight, did not correlate with the level of support. Unfortunately these researchers give no indication of what they see as the limitations (if any) of their research project.

In his commentary on this research paper, Richards (2000) criticises the lack of rigour in this project, while failing to recognise its many achievements. He goes on to argue, unsurprisingly, that 'more research is needed in this area, particularly research which is culturally sensitive'.

The partner

For the purposes of this section I am assuming that the woman's partner is male and that the partner and the baby's father are the same person.

The role of the partner in childbearing has traditionally been viewed merely in terms of the support that he is able to provide for the baby's mother (Bedford & Johnson, 1988). This support has moved on from being merely financial to becoming more wide ranging. Because of this still rather limited role, the partner has tended to feature in the literature only as an adjunct to the mother. That the father also has to establish his own relationship with the baby is increasingly becoming recognised (Bedford & Johnson, 1988). This duality of the partner's role applies throughout the childbearing cycle.

The partner in pregnancy

The role of the partner during pregnancy has attracted little research attention, with the possible exception of his function of supporting his partner's attendance at childbirth education (Nolan & Hicks, 1997; Sullivan-Lyons, 1998: 238). Lewis (1986: 82) has suggested that the picture is 'paradoxical' as the public appearance of being detached serves to conceal intense involvement in the developing relationships.

The partner during labour

The partner is increasingly likely to be in attendance and providing support for the labour and birth. One estimate is that 95% of partners are present at the birth of the couple's baby (MacMillan, 1998). Perhaps for this reason his supportive role at that time has attracted considerable research attention, possibly at the expense of identifying his personal needs (Draper, 1997). That his presence is supportive in nature has tended to be assumed by all concerned. This was assessed in a study (Copstick *et al.*, 1985) which attempted to measure the benefits of the partner's support by using the woman's reports and also her pain ratings. While each woman considered that her partner's presence benefited her through making her pain easier to cope with, the two groups of women showed no significant difference in their pain perception. Thus, the women's experience of labour pain was of equal severity, but appears to have been made more acceptable through his presence.

The partner's supportive role during labour and birth may be enhanced by the woman's high expectations of how he will perform (Ruble *et al.*, 1988). These expectations were investigated in a qualitative study by Somers-Smith (1999). This researcher undertook semi-structured interviews with eight couples, interviewing each member of the couple separately both before and after the birth. The women anticipated that their partner would provide support of a practical nature, such as applying cooling cloths, but his emotional support was expected to be of even greater value. The men found difficulty in defining the specific help which they would be able to offer and tended to fall back on describing their contribution in terms of being a 'familiar face' (Somers-Smith, 1999: 104). This research identified the profound anxieties which men experience in this situation. Their anxieties relate to matters as deep yet as different as the survival of their partner and their own considerable limitations (Somers-Smith, 1999: 104):

'... the extreme of her dying through childbirth which you hear of ...' (Mr C, first interview)
'... I'll be completely shooting in the dark.' (Mr H, first interview)

The men in Somers-Smith's study were found to have come round to the women's expectations of providing more practical forms of support by the time of the labour. These men, like the Hong Kong sample reported by Ip (2000), were surprised when this was rejected and emotional support sought. They were required to provide emotional support of an intensity which they had not expected. Their difficulty in being so intensely supportive was aggravated by their own anxieties and other negative feelings, which they felt they were forced to conceal. On the basis of her data, Somers-Smith (1999: 107) argues that the 'father's needs should be assessed regularly during childbirth'. It is necessary to question whether this recommendation is entirely realistic.

The descriptive retrospective survey by Berry (1988) supports Somers-Smith's findings, by emphasising the negatively stressful nature of the partner's experience of labour. The 40 partners in this study considered that the only time they felt useful was when they were 'coaching' the woman's breathing during the most challenging phase of the labour. The partners found that more of their time in the labour room was spent attempting to conceal their anxieties and worrying about whether they were in the way. Unlike Somers-Smith's recommendation that the partner should be regarded as the midwife's third patient, Berry suggested that education is the answer. An alternative scenario would involve better information on which the couple could base their decision about whether the partner should be present during labour and, if appropriate, better preparation of the partner for his role at that time.

A Finnish study of partners' experiences of childbirth was able to address both the 'pleasure and pride' as well as the 'discomforts' of being present (Vehviläinen-Julkunen & Liukkonen, 1998). This quantitative study involved the application of a questionnaire to partners before the woman and baby were transferred home from the maternity unit. The sample is described as 'non-random', but appears to have been based on convenience. The questionnaire used a Likert-type scale. The important negative feelings experienced by the partners included anxiety, helplessness, uncertainty and worries about their partner coping. An open question asked the partner to recommend changes which would improve midwifery care. Despite being generally happy with care, the partners focused on the need to give more attention, presumably in the form of medication, to control the woman's labour pain. For the partners, having to watch their partner in pain had proved to be one of the most difficult aspects of their experience. This wish to resolve the problem of pain may be related to the partners' discomfort at their own inability to do anything themselves to resolve this problem.

Kitzinger (2000: 4) has described how the partner, through his frustration at his inability to resolve the situation, may seek interventions to 'cure' the pain or to end the labour by 'siding with the obstetrician to help control the little woman'. It has also been suggested that his anxiety may constitute 'a drain on the mother's energy' (Vehviläinen-Julkunen & Liukkonen, 1998). Thus, it may be necessary to reconsider who benefits from the partner being present at the birth, as the support which he is thought to provide may carry with it certain problems (Draper 1998: 237; Odent, 2000). These problems may be experienced not least by the woman in labour.

The partner after the birth

The research literature gives limited attention to the support of the woman by her partner after the birth. The focus tends to be on quite specific aspects of the man's functioning rather than on the relationship. An example of such a specific aspect is his own relationship with his child, which he is likely to be working on throughout the childbearing cycle. This work tends to be emphasised at the expense of his support for the new mother (Bedford & Johnson, 1988; Beail & McGuire, 1982). Alternatively the emphasis may be on specific aspects of the couple's life or relationship, such as breast feeding or their sexuality (Raphael-Leff, 1991: 380).

The changing nature of the couple's relationship after the birth of the first child was investigated by Ruble and colleagues (1988). Data were collected from 670 women in New York using postal questionnaires. The change was usually in the form of a deterioration in the couple's relationship, associated largely with the woman's dissatisfaction. Her less positive feelings compared with pregnancy were attributed more to her unfulfilled expectations of her partner's input and to disillusionment than to the birth of the baby. It is necessary to question whether the pronatalist western society where this research was undertaken fosters unrealistic expectations, which lead all too often to such disillusionment.

In some ways McVeigh's work supports Ruble and colleagues' findings. McVeigh (1997: 173) reports how the woman who is satisfied with the support from her partner is likely to be less stressed, depressed and anxious, and at three months after the birth she is less likely to show overt signs of depression. McVeigh goes on to argue the need for new mothers to actively enlist the support of their partner with routine household responsibilities. This is something which may need to be taught as part of childbirth education, that is, the need to be proactive in negotiating specific and ongoing support. She warns that the new mother should be encouraged not to assume that, as is usually the case, the woman must do everything. This researcher observes that such a change will be neither easy nor intuitive.

While McVeigh's focus was on general aspects of the woman's functioning, there has been more attention given to support in the form of helping the mother provide care for the new baby. Niven (1992: 116) describes how the woman may actually limit the support available to her by controlling the partner's input into baby care. Niven's analysis presents a long term and ongoing picture of the partner often being present but not necessarily supportive. This is likely to be due to the partner being only reactive to the woman's requests and his contribution being little more than a form of 'task allocation'. As shown by the research by Lewis (1986: 88) the mother is perceived as responsible for child care, whereas the father is merely the helper. The tendency has been demonstrated for females to ignore the partner's input. This tendency may carry the danger of becoming a self-fulfilling prophecy. Lewis reported the surprise among his women informants that men may actually be competent in undertaking some child care activities. Some of the men in Lewis' sample considered that they were providing moral support through staying with the woman at difficult times, such as during night feeds. Lewis again highlights the contrast between the public non-involvement and the reality of what he considers to be the men's important contribution.

The baby's grandmother

The need of the new mother for a form of support which has been described as 'mothering' has been identified in a qualitative research project mentioned earlier in the section 'Stress in the post natal period' (Podkolinski, 1998: 222). Podkolinski found that the main sources of the woman's 24 hour support are her partner and her own mother. For one of the women the grandmother's role was stated explicitly to be to 'look after' her (Podkolinski, 1998: 215). The fine line between welcome support and unwanted input was particularly difficult to identify in the context of the woman's mother and her mother-in-law. It was more likely that the mother-in-law would overstep the boundaries of support, only to find herself being accused of 'interference'. The relationship with the grand-mother was found to exert a profound influence on the acceptability of her involvement; thus a grandmother could be described in terms of being 'too dogmatic' with the result that she became 'more of a hindrance'.

For first time mothers the security of knowing that there would be someone at home with experience and with whom a trusting relationship existed, was para-mount. Thus one woman reported that although 'really scared', due to her mother's presence 'I knew I'd be safe' (Podkolinski, 1998: 219). Podkolinski concludes that although the 'mothering' role traditionally undertaken by the grandmother remains crucial, because of societal changes it is now more likely to be offered by the professional.

This conclusion contradicts the rose-tinted picture presented, based largely on personal experience, by Downe (1998). Her list of benefits of the grandmother's input begins with the special relationship derived from the genetic bond. That the young mother is able to leave her child with the grandmother with a clear con-science results from this common background. The psychological work on the mother-daughter relationship during pregnancy is described as one of the joys of parenthood. These joys are further exemplified in the pleasurable reactions and reassuring support of the new grandmother. Downe's underlying assumption is that 'your mother is there for you' (Downe, 1998: 682).

Unfortunately, much of the literature on grandparenting (Walsh, 1989; McCullough & Rutenberg, 1989) makes assumptions, like Downe, that grand-parents are 'in later life' and, hence, constantly available. This assumption may not be supported by demographic evidence and emerged in a study of the support of families with a very low birth weight baby (McHaffie, 1996). This study found that the babies' grandparents ranged in age from their 'thirties to the sixties'. Similarly, writers who assume that grandparents have nothing to do other than be grandparents may be being less than realistic. My observation while working with new mothers leads me to believe that many grandmothers are not available to provide support for the new mother because they are young enough still to be employed on a full time basis. My observations may serve to endorse those made by Podkolinski.

Another research project which focused on the support offered around the time of the birth involved 86 family units (Hansen & Jacob, 1992). These researchers identified the difficulty which the grandparents may experience in recognising the extent to which childcare ideas and practices have changed since they first became parents. Although this time may be only 16 to 20 years, ideas about childcare can change markedly. Such difficulty with providing relevant support is likely to limit what the grandparents are able to offer the new parents. A variety of other factors may further affect the grandparents' support, including geographical proximity, ethnicity and culture. Hanson and Jacob found that the timing of the grand-parental support was likely to be deferred by the new parents who soon realised, however, that their expectations of becoming a strictly nuclear family were less than realistic and the support of grandparents was eventually welcomed.

Compared with the beneficial role of the grandmother which emerged in the research by Podkolinski and, to a lesser extent, in that by Hansen and Jacob, Kitzinger (1978) presents a more negative view. She focuses on the potential for conflict between the mother and the grandmother, the relatively low status of the grandmother in industrialised societies and the coping strategies which have evolved in a number of societies to defuse conflict.

The grandparents of very low birth weight babies were found by McHaffie (1996) to be crucial in providing both emotional and practical support to the new parents. Of particular significance was the shared recognition of the 'high priority' (McHaffie, 1996: 251) of the new baby in the parents' lives. The variability in the appropriateness of the support offered by the grandparents, as mentioned already in the work of Downe and Kitzinger, was examined. This evaluation of the various grandparents' contributions showed the maternal grandmothers scoring highest and the grandfathers lowest. McHaffie (1996: 252) found that informational support from grandparents was the least welcome, probably due to the 'very specialised situation' in which the baby was being treated.

The role of the grandmother which has been recounted as applying on a longer term basis is that of the 'watchdog' (Troll, 1983). This role may be required around the time of the birth as much as at any other time. The essential feature of the role is that the grandmother is able to be present and to give the benefit of her experience only if and when it is needed and sought. Thus the grandmother carries what may be termed a 'watching brief', which allows her freedom from her young family. This freedom continues until the family is in need of her assistance, at which point she is able to step in to help. Thus, Troll observes that the grandmother 'can often appear uninvolved' (Troll, 1983: 64), but her involvement only becomes apparent as and when it is required.

Conclusion

The stress of childbearing has been shown to have implications which are both wide ranging and long lasting. The extent to which social support is able to remedy such negative effects is less than certain. In spite of this uncertainty, the need for support at this challenging time is undisputed. Additionally, those research projects involving the provision of support have clearly indicated the satisfaction of the women who have been recipients of support. The support has been shown to be provided by a range of personnel as well as partners, family and relatives, the significance of whom should not be underestimated. One of the personnel whose supportive role has not yet been examined is the midwife, and this is addressed in the next chapter.

Chapter 4
Supportive midwifery care

In the earlier chapters the effects of social support in more general situations have been examined. In this chapter I further adjust the focus to examine in detail the support which is provided in childbearing by one particular occupational group – the midwife. Because health care is usually organised according to a more or less formal system of care, it is now necessary to consider whether and how midwifery care offers support within that system. This is necessary in part due to the increasing realisation of the finite nature of resources available to the health care system. Policy makers and care providers are thus being required to account for their use of those resources.

Many aspects of the care of the childbearing woman are being subjected to scrutiny in order to justify the allocation of resources. Efficiency and effectiveness are two of the criteria widely used to warrant resource allocation to particular services. Efficiency has been defined as 'how well one does something', and effectiveness as 'how successfully an aim is achieved' (Paton, 1995: 31).The other criteria often used include acceptability, sustainability and equity (Garcia & Campbell, 1997: 14). In this chapter the focus is on the effectiveness of supportive midwifery care as one of the fundamental characteristics of the maternity services. Having previously reviewed the benefits of support, I am here assuming that one of the main aims of the midwife is to provide appropriately supportive care for the childbearing woman. Thus, in this chapter I scrutinise the research literature in order to assess whether the midwife does provide support and, if so, whether that support has been shown to be of benefit to the woman and to her baby.

Before examining the research and the findings on the effectiveness of supportive midwifery care, it may be helpful to compare the methods and criteria which have been employed by researchers in order to investigate this phenomenon. I next look at developments in care which have approached supportive care at discrete points in the woman's childbearing cycle. Finally, I address the strategies suggested, researched and/or implemented with a view to improving the woman's complete childbearing experience.

Evaluative methods

In contemplating the benefits or otherwise of supportive midwifery care, the research literature shows us that there are a number of methods which may be utilised to investigate it. Each of the various methods has its own disciples. Because of the ensuing debates about their relative merits it is necessary to examine closely some of the more frequently-used approaches and methods.

Evidence

That midwifery should be a research-based profession has been recommended and sought since the Briggs Report (1972). More recently, in the course of our medical colleagues' attempts to put their house in order, the requirements have been raised to aim for evidence-based practice (EBP). These attempts followed Cochrane's original plea for a sound research base to medical practice and his appropriately scathing criticisms of obstetricians' lack of any such base (Cochrane, 1972). The cornerstone of EBP is the randomised controlled trial (RCT) which, if undertaken suitably rigorously, is widely recognised as the 'gold standard' for evidence on which to build practice. The status of EBP has been confirmed by a government-backed innovation, known as 'clinical governance', of which EBP is one of the bases (Scally & Donaldson, 1998). This innovation may be little more than a knee-jerk reaction to the problems encountered by our medical colleagues with their public image (McSherry & Haddock, 1999). According to its advocates, the clinical governance framework is intended to create a care environment which 'supports good quality care based on evidence and sound judgement' (Galbraith, 1998: 3).

While recognising the need for improvement in the research basis of some midwives' practice, criticisms have been articulated (Page, 1996). The requirement for all midwifery practice to be based on evidence is theoretically sound, but the implementation has been 'complicated' (Webster *et al.*, 1999: 2). The initial criticisms and complications of midwives' application of EBP were summarised in the following terms:

(1) Midwives have always practised this way (Walsh, 1996)
(2) The evidence is unrelated to the real world (Hardy & Mulhall, 1994)
(3) It is not feasible for RCTs to be the only source on which to base clinical decisions, as not all situations or interventions have been evaluated (Walsh, 1996; Page, 1997)
(4) Midwives may reject attempts to limit their autonomy by management regimes perceived as authoritarian and are then labelled as the 'clinical freedom fighters' (Page, 1997)
(5) The reductionist approach to care makes no allowance for the intuition, values, consumer's opinions and gut feelings which serve to make up caring practice (Sackett *et al.*, 1996)
(6) The limited time which practitioners have available makes it difficult for them to always check the research report before an intervention. Thus, the crucially important context in which the research was undertaken may be missed (Walsh, 1996; Page, 1997).

With increasing knowledge of EBP, more profound criticisms have been articulated. Clarke (1999) discusses the relative salience of the different forms of knowledge on which health care is based. She argues that EBP is leading to an overvaluing of 'scientific' knowledge with a corresponding devaluation of the human aspects of knowledge. Clarke (1999: 91) depicts a hierarchy of knowledge, in which the softer, more experience-based forms are relegated to a lowly position 'at the bottom of the league table'. She considers that a re-evaluation is urgently needed. Thus, for a health care provider to be able to make a sound decision, far more than just research evidence is required. The decision-making process should also be informed by 'personal instincts and intuition, listening to our patients rather than only to research literature' (Clarke, 1999: 92).

Clarke recommends that greater introspection would assist the health care provider to decide what sources of information may most appropriately be used in a given situation. This recommendation requires that, in order to decide not to use it, the practitioner must be aware of the existence of research evidence, in addition to the human sources of knowledge. Thus, the challenge to the practitioner of accessing, evaluating and assimilating the mass of evidence persists. For this reason, in examining the literature on supportive midwifery practice, I will draw on a range of both more human as well as more scientific research methods.

Audit

Unlike research in the maternity area, audit differs in that it has not been subjected to the scrutiny of a research ethics committee (Maresh, 1999). Occasionally, one may be forgiven for wondering whether this is the only difference. In this chapter I attempt to use only those audits which fit the more acceptable criteria:

(1)   Well-localised functionally and/or geographically
(2)   A continuing activity
(3)   Having measurable objectives to ensure relevant comparisons
(4)   Intending that an action will ensue, such as a change in service provision.
                    (Brandom, 1996; Rees, 1997: 8; Campbell, 1997: 6)

The crucial role of the clinical environment becomes apparent in the three aspects in which audit is traditionally undertaken, that is with its focus on structure or process or outcome. While the process is most frequently addressed by audit, it is this aspect which is least likely to be satisfactorily audited (Walsh, 1999: 430). The problem, according to Walsh, is that the audit loop is unlikely to be completely closed. By this, he means that guidelines are set and data are collected, but strategies to correct any shortfall may not be implemented and there is no evaluation of any change in practice when it is implemented. Thus, the audit process is effectively stalled, and the audit cycle is unable to proceed to develop into the continuing audit spiral which leads to improvement in health care (Maresh, 1999: 137).

Although numerical approaches are often assumed to be fundamental to audit,

Maresh (1999: 140) maintains that this is not necessarily the case. He argues that obtaining the woman's views about her care is an 'alternative method of auditing maternal morbidity' (Maresh, 1999: 140). Such data may be obtained qualitatively rather than quantitatively in order to learn of the woman's perspective on her pregnancy outcome.

Some of the problems inherent in audit manifested themselves in a study of a change in maternity care based on the recommendations of the *Changing Childbirth* report (Beake *et al.*, 1998; DoH, 1993). One example is that the demarcation between audit, which addresses ongoing practice, and research, which features a new intervention, appears to have become blurred in the context of this study. Thus, my opening criticism of audit may still be justified, rather than being the historical problem to which Walsh (1999: 430) refers. Another of the problems which Beake and colleagues encountered in the course of their audit related to data collection. They relied on the woman's medical case notes to provide the data which they planned to utilise for audit purposes. These auditors found that the instruments which they were using as data collection tools had, in practice, been developed for quite a different purpose, that is, as records of care. Thus, these researchers were able to draw only limited conclusions about the effects of the woman-centred intervention which they introduced.

Evaluative criteria

As mentioned in the introduction to this chapter, a number of criteria have been suggested as indicators of the effectiveness of supportive midwifery care, not least the 'three Cs' – continuity, choice and control (Hundley *et al.*, 1997). Attempts have been made to discredit the 'three Cs' as indicators of the woman's satisfaction with her maternity care (Young, 1999: 14). In spite of this, Young maintains that by considering these indicators it may be possible to find out more accurately what the woman is seeking and gaining from her childbearing experience. Thus, they are considered here as criteria which may be used to facilitate evaluation.

Continuity

Continuity as one of the 'three Cs' has had 'a bad press' for a number of reasons, some of which are outlined by Waldenström (1998). One of these reasons relates to uncertainty about whether the continuity refers to the person providing the care or to the philosophy which underpins that care. Another reason is that continuity may be sought through the farce of the pregnant woman meeting, and supposedly coming to 'know', up to eight midwives during her pregnancy (Young, 1999: 16); the intention is that, when in labour, the woman will be attended by a 'known' midwife. It is my observation that attempts to ensure that the woman meets all of the eight midwives become frenetic to the point of being counterproductive as the time for the birth draws near. It would also be difficult to argue that having met a midwife on one occasion constitutes 'knowing' her. Perhaps unsurprisingly, Young maintains that he as a general practitioner is in a better position to provide continuity of care, even to the point of inter-generational continuity (Young, 1999: 16). He does condescend to admit, however, that the general practitioner is 'unlikely' to provide care right through labour.

Continuity has assumed greater significance due to the increasing fragmentation of ante natal care. Fragmentation is difficult to disentangle from the effects of the medicalisation of maternity care. A supportive relationship during labour is thought to be easily developed following regular and frequent contact during pregnancy. Such a relationship may, however, be more elusive if the woman and the midwife are strangers.

The research projects which have focused on continuity of care have, inevitably, involved care by midwives (Flint *et al.*, 1989; Rowley *et al.*, 1995). These studies have been criticised because of their inability to distinguish continuity of care from midwifery care (Hodnett, 2000b: 5). This criticism is hardly valid, as the likelihood of any other occupational group having either the skills or the inclination to provide continuity of care is remote. This critic's suggestion of the need for a study of continuity of physician care is less than realistic. What these studies have achieved, however, is to distinguish and show the benefits of continuity of midwifery care compared with the routine, fragmented and multidisciplinary variety.

This conclusion is endorsed by a Swedish study which showed that the identity of the individual midwife providing care in labour was not the woman's prime concern (Waldenström, 1998). This study, which was part of a large RCT, indicated that the woman's first priority was the nature of her care. The second most important factor was the environment for the birth. The third factor was that the woman should have known the same team of midwives throughout her childbearing experience. Thus, it is clear that it is the care and the shared philosophy underpinning that care which matter more to the childbearing woman than 'knowing' the individual carer.

Choice

Summarised as 'the new shibboleth of maternity political correctness' (Mander 1993: 23), choice may also have been relegated to the realms of illusion. It is difficult to ascertain whether the scope for the childbearing woman to make real choices has changed since Richards wrote his scathing and ground-breaking paper in 1982. That the situation has not improved is supported by the less than wholehearted welcome extended to the 'Informed Choice' leaflets (Oliver *et al.*, 1996). This innovation, which was intended to provide the childbearing woman with evidence on which to base the choices open to her during pregnancy, was welcomed by midwives. The reception by other health care personnel, however, was lukewarm, with doubts about the validity of the evidence tinged with anxiety about organisational and professional issues.

The professionals appear to continue to be reluctant to provide the woman with the necessary information on which to base her decisions. This reluctance threatens the woman's ability to take full advantage of the choices with which she is presented. The limited availability of research evidence on maternity issues has been highlighted in the debate on evidence-based practice (see the earlier section 'Evidence'). That the evidence which is available is not being disseminated appropriately throws into doubt much of the well-intentioned rhetoric which followed the Winterton Report (1992). This example may serve as a reminder of the importance of communication as a precursor to information-giving which, in turn, is crucial to the making of sound choices.

Control

The terms 'choice' and 'control' are not necessarily synonymous, even though the close interrelationship between them may suggest otherwise. In their important study Green and colleagues (1990) investigated the relationship between these concepts. They concluded that choice facilitates control and that an absence of choice implies absence of control. The corollary, of which these researchers warned, is that in some people and in some circumstances the presence of choice may serve to decrease control by engendering anxiety. Thus, a complex picture emerges as these researchers showed that control is not a unidimensional phenomenon. Further, it became apparent that the woman's needs for control cannot be generalised. The assumptions so beloved of health care personnel may not have a sound basis. Green's study showed that a woman's wish for control may not correlate with, for example, her attendance at childbirth education, her socio-economic class, her occupation, or her previous childbearing experience. Green and colleagues warn that, at least in the context of control, stereotyping may be less than helpful.

This examination of control has been moved forward by other researchers, whose work suggests that environmental factors may also affect the woman's ability to assume control of her childbearing experience. This has been shown to apply, first, to the effects of the woman's strictly physical environment when the woman chooses to give birth at home (Spitzer, 1995; Morison *et al.*, 1998). Other less tangible aspects of the environment have also been shown to influence the woman's ability to assume control; for example, Weaver (1998) suggests that the carer's personal and occupational experience may also feature in the control equation. In even broader terms, personal relationships with staff have been described as being fundamental to the woman's sense of control (Green *et al.*, 1990). Thus, the concept of control may prove to be both interactive and dynamic (Weaver, 1998: 90).

Control has been shown to influence outcomes, first, on a short term basis; this emerged in the finding that higher expectations correlate strongly and positively with higher satisfaction (Green *et al.*, 1990). In the long term, Simkin (1992) has shown that a sense of control carries benefits lasting for 20 years. Kitzinger (1992), on the other hand, reminds us that the reverse also applies and that the negative feelings associated with a lack of control during childbearing may persist for 50 to 60 years.

Quality

As well as the three specific aspects of maternity care discussed above, the 'three Cs', evaluation of the quality of maternity services tends to utilise mortality or serious morbidity data (Wiegers *et al.*, 1996). These criteria may be less than appropriate in the context of uncomplicated childbearing. For this reason more relevant quality assessment tools are being sought. An example of one of these instruments which measures more generally the effectiveness of midwifery care is the pro-forma for monitoring and managing midwifery quality, developed by Martin-Hirsch and Wright (1998).

Satisfaction

The assessment of the woman's satisfaction with her maternity or midwifery care is fraught with problems (Currell, 1996). This may be due, at least in part, to uncertainty about what comprises satisfaction; this is exemplified in Currell's (1996: 9) writing when she regards satisfaction and continuity as synonymous. Uncertainties such as this are thought to be responsible for the limited published evaluations of the recent crop of new maternity care schemes (Wraight *et al.*, 1993). It is necessary to question whether this sorry picture is caused by the client's dissatisfaction, the lack of any evaluation or the midwife's well-recognised reluctance to venture into print (Mander, 1995). The difficulties of evaluating satisfaction have been recognised since Lumley in 1985 demonstrated that soft outcomes present really hard problems to researchers. These difficulties relate not only to the nature of the data collection instrument, but also to when it is applied and the person who applies it. Additionally, difficulty may be encountered in distinguishing the woman's satisfaction with her new baby from her feelings about her experience of birth (Currell, 1996).

An example of these difficulties is a satisfaction study which was undertaken in Canada when maternity care there was still widely and intensively medicalised (Séguin *et al.*, 1989). On the basis of a 52.4% response rate the researchers were perhaps surprisingly able to conclude that there is a high level of satisfaction with health care (Séguin *et al.*, 1989: 112). It may be that subsequent events have presented a more accurate comment on Canadian women's satisfaction with medicalised maternity care (see Chapter 2).

Some of the methodological difficulties encountered by the Canadian study were resolved in a large study (*n* = 1299) undertaken in Glasgow by Shields and colleagues (1998). The study comprised an RCT in which randomisation resulted in 648 women allocated to midwife managed care and 651 women to standard shared care (Turnbull *et al.*, 1996). This study, again, showed the women's satisfaction, but this was significantly higher throughout the childbearing experience in the group who received the intervention of midwife-managed care. The areas of satisfaction identified related to relationships with staff, information giving, choices and decisions and social support.

It is probably only right that satisfaction as an indicator of the effectiveness of midwifery care should focus more on the experience of the woman than the midwife. The relationship of these two phenomena, however, may not be as clear or as simple as assumed. Sandall (1998) reports her research into how well the midwife copes with the challenge of new working arrangements. This study showed that, although midwives are more satisfied by offering a midwifery service which is of a higher standard, the hazards of the longer working hours which they invest may outweigh the benefits.

Reid and colleagues (1997) advance a form of conspiracy theory to explain these developments. These authors argue that women, on the one hand, are being misled into believing that a service is available, when in fact it is dependent on the goodwill of the midwifery staff. On the other hand, midwives are being inveigled into providing a high quality service on a shoestring. Thus, the midwife may be forced to choose whether she will jeopardise her health by being involved, or her career by declining involvement.

Other criteria

This list of criteria which may be employed to evaluate midwifery care has focused on those which are likely to impinge on the support offered to the woman. Clearly other criteria may be and have been used. Because of the resource-conscious nature of the current health care system, economic criteria are increasingly likely to feature (Hundley *et al.*, 1995; Twaddle & Young, 1999). In midwifery care, as in other forms of health care (see the section 'Access and equity' in Chapter 2), certain fundamental ethical principles of provision apply, such as accessibility and equity (Garcia & Campbell, 1997). Clinical outcomes, as mentioned earlier, are important considerations, but safety is becoming more and more difficult to measure as serious morbidity and mortality become rarer (Currell, 1996).

Support in innovative midwifery care

A backlash against the obstetric excesses of the 1970s resulted in a groundswell seeking changes in the culture of childbearing in the late 1980s (Garcia *et al.*, 1990). Together with midwives, consumer groups were sufficiently vocal to persuade policy makers and others to introduce innovations to change the traditional, or at least longstanding, system of maternity care. The Winterton Committee, although possibly not entirely objective in its collection of evidence, produced a report which broke new ground by clearly requiring that the woman's needs should be central to maternity care provision (Winterton Report, 1992). The government, in response, set up an expert committee to review policy and make recommendations; in England these recommendations took the form of the report *Changing Childbirth* (1993). One of the major bases of this report was the implementation of the Winterton Committee's plan to dismantle the 'medical model' of maternity care (*Changing Childbirth*, 1993: 1). These authoritative recommendations served to fuel the demand for change by building on existing innovations and facilitating others. These developments have encouraged a re-examination by midwives and others of the role of the midwife and, particularly, her role in providing support to the childbearing woman. Some of these developments have approached particular aspects of the woman's care, whereas others have sought to address her complete childbearing experience. The more complete approaches will be examined first.

The 'Know Your Midwife' scheme

The first authoritative study of the phalanx of novel midwifery care schemes was the 'Know Your Midwife' (KYM) project based in St George's hospital in London (Flint *et al.*, 1989). This randomised controlled trial sought and achieved scientific credibility, perhaps at the expense of the assessment of the 'softer' outcomes. Continuity of care was the explicit aim of this midwifery team, so outcomes such as client satisfaction and the woman's perceptions of being supported featured negligibly, if at all. Interestingly, the midwives' ability to provide effective support for each other featured much more prominently. The team of four midwives was highly committed and motivated. This RCT demonstrated that, over a two year period, care could be provided for 500 'low risk' women with better continuity, reduced medical intervention and lower episiotomy rates. This high standard, in terms of research method and results, has been achieved by few of the other team midwifery schemes which blossomed in the wake of the KYM findings (Wraight *et al.*, 1993).

Team midwifery

In a UK survey of the introduction of team midwifery schemes, Wraight and colleagues (1993) identified the enthusiasm which the KYM findings aroused among midwives and midwife managers. Unfortunately a large proportion of the schemes which were established on the basis of this enthusiasm lacked the driving force which ensured the success of KYM. Thus, they soon foundered. The reasons for their foreshortened survival and limited success include uncertainty about the 'ideal size' for a midwifery team which aims to balance the woman's needs against the demands on the midwife. Although enthusiasm and commitment may have been sufficient to initiate these schemes, they were often inadequate to overcome the day-to-day problems of ensuring cover for wards as well as providing intrapartum care and meeting community obligations. The serious implications of the massive changes in the midwife's level of responsibility may also have been underestimated during the planning of these innovative schemes (Todd *et al.*, 1998).

In spite of the difficulties which the midwife is likely to encounter in a system of team midwifery, the woman is likely to be more satisfied by this organisation of care (Tinkler & Quinney, 1998). On the basis of a 'pilot' study involving 68 women, Tinkler and Quinney identified the crucial contribution of the supportive relationship between the woman and midwife. These researchers found that the woman sought an equal input into decisions relating to the offering and nature of the midwife's support. Thus timely support would be welcomed, as also would support which did not jeopardise the woman's autonomy. Support which was perceived as 'dominating' or 'interfering' was compared unfavourably by the women with 'enabling' support (Tinkler & Quinney, 1998: 34). The woman's preparedness to relinquish her control in certain situations demonstrated the extent to which the nature of the relationship was determined by the woman.

In her uncompromising assessment of a team midwifery scheme in Oxford, Bower (1993) considers the implications of teams for both the woman and the midwife. The scheme clearly demonstrated benefits and costs for both parties. Bower's overall impression is, as mentioned earlier in the section on 'Satisfaction', that the advantages to the women are provided at the cost of the midwife's humane working conditions. Her examples include midwives being called to work on their days off and the 'impact on the personal life of each midwife'. Perhaps as a result of these costs, the team scheme, though initially expanded, soon ceased to grow.

Such uncertainty about the future of team midwifery is also reflected in the work of Hart and colleagues (1999). These researchers found that, in their evaluation, the woman was less concerned about continuity of care during labour than continuity of support during the antepartum period. Their comparison between traditional maternity care and team care showed equivalent high levels of satisfaction with both systems. Without detailing this scheme's economic assessment, Hart and colleagues indicate that the other reason for its uncertain future is due to a lack of evidence to persuade the trust 'to invest in the future of the scheme' (Hart *et al.*, 1999: 577).

One-to-one midwifery

The prospective comparative demonstration project undertaken in London by Page and colleagues sought to operationalise the *Changing Childbirth* recommendations (McCourt *et al.*, 1998). The specific foci were woman-centred care and continuity of carer. The project aimed to allocate one midwife to each childbearing woman, and care was provided and planned by that midwife (McCourt & Page, 1996). The 'neighbourhood basis' of the study prevented the randomisation of the childbearing women into groups. But choices were available to the woman about the place where care would be provided (hospital or community) and about the discipline of the lead professional (midwife, GP or obstetrician). The limited duration of the project resulted in a study group comprising 728 women and a control group of 675 women.

This project showed that continuity of carer was sought by the woman and that, in labour, the woman prefers care to be by a known midwife. Particularly valued by the woman in the intervention group was the high level of constant support while in labour. This support was associated with a significant reduction in the woman's use of 'epidural anaesthesia' (Page *et al.*, 1999). Lower rates of perineal damage and shorter second stage of labour were also identified. The women in the intervention group linked the greater midwifery support with better information-giving. This much-appreciated intrapartum support was available to the woman continuously from the time of the home assessment when labour was beginning. Comparison may be appropriate with the somewhat less optimistic study by Hart and colleagues (1999) mentioned above.

The researchers were able to follow up women who did not respond to the self completion questionnaires. This was by conducting interviews with them. McCourt and colleagues (1998) found that 'disadvantaged' women were over-represented among these non-responders. These interview data draw attention to one of the most serious contradictions in the UK maternity care system – that the system is least able to provide support to those women whose need for support is greatest.

Midwife-managed care

In Glasgow a form of team midwifery care was introduced experimentally in the Midwifery Development Unit (MDU) (McGinley *et al.*, 1995). The aim of the project was to provide continuity of both care and carer. The providers of care are sometimes referred to as 'a team of 20 midwives', although this number may be reduced to 'a small group of midwives' (McGinley, 1995: 362). The eventual decision to adopt a caseload system of care resulted in each woman being allocated a named midwife. The self-rostering pattern of off-duty, though, meant that there was no certainty that a woman's named midwife would be on duty when she went into labour. Additionally, even if the named midwife were on duty, there was a 50% chance that she would be working somewhere other than in the labour ward. Because of the shift pattern for the MDU midwife in the labour ward, three associate midwives were also nominated. Such a limited continuity of carer, McGinley and colleagues (1995) emphasise, requires the explicit implementation of a common philosophy of care in order to facilitate continuity of care.

The RCT which was undertaken to evaluate the system of care in the MDU involved 1299 women, of whom 648 were randomised to midwife-managed care and 651 to the standard form of 'shared care' (Turnbull *et al.*, 1996; Shields *et al.*, 1998). This trial showed that both groups of women were generally satisfied with their care. The MDU woman, though, was more likely to be satisfied with her relationships with staff, with information giving, with choices and decisions and with social support. Although the MDU woman was also likely to be more satisfied with her care throughout her childbearing experience, the difference was most marked when the care differed most, that is during the ante natal period and during the hospital-based post natal care. This observation applied as much to the woman's experience of social support as it did to the other relatively 'soft' outcomes which were investigated (Shields *et al.*, 1998: 89).

The possibility of midwife-managed care meeting the deficiencies in support highlighted in the work of McCourt and colleagues (1998), mentioned above, emerges in a more recent account of the Glasgow MDU (Turnbull *et al.*, 1999). This report shows that, in spite of the large numbers of midwives in the 'team', and in spite of the off-duty system, the MDU woman invariably encountered fewer carers than the woman receiving shared care. This form of continuity of carer was particularly important in terms of the MDU midwives' ability to ensure consistency of advice to the woman. Thus, continuity of care also ensued. These encouraging outcomes were achieved in spite of the large proportion (39–42%) of the women who resided in a neighbourhood classified on a seven point scale as least affluent. In this way McCourt and colleagues' (1998) finding of the least support available to the most vulnerable may not be insuperable.

Personal caseload midwifery

Another innovative system of midwifery care which attempted to implement the recommendations of the *Changing Childbirth* (1993) report also focused on providing woman-centred care and better continuity of care (Morgan *et al.*, 1998). These researchers sought to compare the perceptions of the women who had been involved in two different forms of midwifery group practice. These schemes comprised a shared caseload practice and a personal caseload practice. The evaluation was made on the basis of the likelihood of the woman seeing the same midwife during pregnancy, the likelihood that a midwife she had met before would attend her birth and the woman's preferences in relation to continuity and satisfaction with her care. Personal caseload practice achieved better continuity ante natally and this was associated with greater satisfaction, even though a smaller number of women had met the midwife who attended the birth. On the basis of these findings the researchers conclude that continuity of carer is not directly associated with the woman's satisfaction with her care. More important than continuity is the supportiveness of care, its consistency, the standard of communication and the woman's input into decision-making.

Independent midwifery

A further form of midwifery practice which may offer more effective continuity of care, and the associated supportive relationship, is independent midwifery. My own limited personal experience of independent practice convinces me that this form of practice is more complete and, like Sidney (1999), I consider that every effort should be made to preserve it. Evaluation of independent practice is sadly lacking, possibly due to the small numbers of independent midwives. In her research project, Demilew (1996) found that for the one year studied, 41 midwives in England had notified their intention to practise independently. Of these, Demilew was able to interview 32. As well as demographic data and reasons for practising independently, this study identified the independent midwife's perception of her role. The recurring theme through these midwives' accounts is the midwife's ability to support the woman to achieve the birth experience which she is seeking.

Adverse publicity due to highly publicised legal cases involving independent midwives and changes in insurance status have combined to threaten the future of independent midwifery. This publicity has presented the negative view of this form of practice. An entirely different view is presented by the account of the work of the South East London Midwifery Group through their statistics (SELMG, 1994). These midwives compare the caesarean rate for the women they attend (6%) with the local rate in standard NHS care (27%). Of the women booked with SELMG, 75% gave birth at home compared with a national average of between 1% and 2%. This group's perinatal mortality rate was 7.7 (per 1000 total births) compared with 8.8 for England and Wales (ONS, 1996). The breast feeding rate among SELMG clients was 95%, compared with a maximum rate of 65% for England and Wales (HEBS, 1995).

It is necessary to recognise that the SELMG data represent the findings from a self-selected sample. It may be that the real indicators of the implications of independent midwifery practice lie somewhere between these ideal figures and the highly publicised 'cases'. It is necessary to conclude, though, that the possibility of a woman giving birth supported by a midwife who is really known to her appears greater with a group like SELMG than with the other schemes which have been reported.

Community intervention

I have been considering the provision of supportive midwifery care throughout the woman's childbearing experience. Those schemes which have been described so far have comprised an *alternative* to some standard form of care. It is now necessary to focus on a form of midwifery care which has been provided to *complement* that standard maternity care (Davies, 1997a). In an area which would now be said to demonstrate a high level of 'social exclusion', a midwifery intervention was introduced in an attempt to reduce the high perinatal mortality rates. The intervention was planned to offer extra care to vulnerable women. The four midwives provided cover for each other and each woman was seen mainly by one midwife. These contacts happened in the woman's home, in the local drop-in centre and in unplanned street encounters as well as through other planned activities. The midwives interpreted 'extra care' broadly, to include activities, such as cooking, which were only tangentially, if at all, related to maternity matters. The midwives' philosophy was that 'primary health care should be neighbourhood based' (Davies, 1997a: 110). The midwives were required to work hard to overcome resistance, which was partly from the community but also from local medical personnel.

In the account of her evaluation of this project, Evans (1997) details the measurable benefits, such as significantly better attendance at childbirth education. The reduction in the number of pre-term births compared with the control group reinforces the suggestion made previously (see Chapter 3) that supportive interventions affect clinical outcomes. The women's satisfaction with their 'extra care' emerges clearly from Evans' discussion of her findings.

Evans (1997) contrasts the usual assumptions, about the working-class woman being well supported by a network of family and friends, with the reality of this woman's life. The one-to-one relationship with the project midwife was particularly appreciated because of the women 'having very few supportive relationships in their lives' (Evans, 1997: 125). The foundation for this support was in the presence of the midwives in the community (Davies, 1997b: 53), although some of the menfolk exhibited behaviour which indicated their perceptions of being threatened by these developments. Despite such opposition the sessions which began as parentcraft classes (Davies, 1997b: 52) developed into and continued as self-support groups. These sessions were sufficiently popular for the new mother to attend and require 'the classes' to evolve after the birth (Davies, 1990: 30). The changes which engendered these positive developments were not solely among the women in the community, whose confidence in their own ability was enhanced. Davies (1997b: 61) recognises the work which was required of the midwife in order to support the mother to achieve such changes. The basis of the midwife's supportive role, Davies maintains, lies in her acceptance of the mother for who she actually is.

Supportive midwifery care at discrete points in the childbearing cycle

As well as the approaches which have been described already to provide effective supportive care throughout the woman's childbearing experience, other schemes have sought to address specific problems at certain well-defined points in the woman's experience. Clearly labour constitutes one of these well-defined points. Because of its significance to all involved, as well as to the researcher, the role of support in labour is addressed in the next chapter (Chapter 5).

During the pregnancy

The maternity services in general and ante natal care in particular have long been the subject of criticism for their lack of humanity (MoH, 1961). A scheme which sought to change this by providing better continuity in community maternity care has long been established in Sighthill, Edinburgh (McKee, 1984). While the effects on midwifery practice and on measurable outcomes are well recounted in the literature (Staines, 1986), the effects on the woman's experience are less clear. It is possible that this omission may relate to the priorities of the early 1970s when this scheme was established.

The development of the supportive role of the midwife during pregnancy is traced by two Swedish researchers (Hildingsson & Häggström, 1999). This qualitative study recruited seven midwives who worked in five different ante natal clinics. Each of the midwives was happy to talk about the support she was able to provide and, especially, about the importance of this aspect of the midwife's role. The midwife encountered more difficulty, however, in explaining how she learnt about providing support and what it involved. It was often necessary for the midwife to resort to speaking about support in terms of its being 'instinctive' or describing her perception of the need as based on 'ethical reflections and situational insight'. Surprisingly for a country as affluent as Sweden, the women in this study were relatively unsupported by menfolk and family. This factor served to require an even more supportive role of the midwife.

The complexity of the midwife's support emerged in the accounts of it being an indirect activity. This means that the support is not just for the woman herself but involves the midwife's identification and nurturing of the existing resources which she may have available to her, but does not fully utilise. Examples of these indirect activities include empowering the woman through helping to build up her self-esteem and also by encouraging her to act as her own advocate for herself.

The term which Hildingsson and Häggström use to summarise the supportive activities of the midwife is one which may be regarded by some as less than appropriate due to its association with reduced autonomy. This term is 'mothering', which has been used in different ways to describe the relationship between the woman and her carers. These researchers use 'mothering' to indicate an empowering by the more experienced woman, the midwife, for the new mother. It also carries with it the sense of the more experienced woman acting as an exemplar or role model of the 'good mother'. This aspect of the mothering role assumed particular significance in the Swedish context where families were described as often being dysfunctional or fractured. A further sense of the indirect input of the midwife emerges in the logical extension of this exemplar role. In this way the midwife acts more specifically as a 'mother' to the woman in order to facilitate her ability to nurture her baby. This indirect intervention is summarised in terms of 'mothering the mother to mother her baby'.

In the maternity unit after the birth

As mentioned in Chapter 3 in the section 'Support in the post natal period' some forms of support to reduce psychological morbidity have not been accepted uncritically or universally. Alexander (1998) has appropriately criticised the widely and often incorrectly used term 'debriefing'. An example of this incorrect usage may be found in a study of post natal psychological morbidity, where it was used rather loosely (Lavender & Walkinshaw, 1998). These researchers defined it in terms of 'a psychological intervention intended to reduce the psychological morbidity that arises after exposure to a traumatic event ... the intervention did not include in-depth questioning' (Lavender & Walkinshaw, 1998: 216). The authors emphasise the strong element of support which was a feature of the intervention. Randomisation of eligible women and the listening and discussion intervention were completed in the post natal ward. The interviews were all undertaken by one midwife who had not received any special preparation for her role. A questionnaire and anxiety/depression assessment instrument were posted to each woman three weeks later. The intervention group included 58 women, compared with the control group of 56.

The assessed differences in the psychological morbidity of the two groups were found to be highly significant (p < 0.0001). The researchers admit to uncertainty about the reasons for this finding. They suggest that these differences might be due to the participants in the two arms of the trial not being 'blinded' or to the instrument used not being appropriate to the post natal period. In spite of these potentially confounding uncertainties, the researchers confidently assert that the support provided through this midwifery intervention does serve to enhance psychological well-being.

Surprisingly, the commentary on this research report (Wessely, 1998) accepts the authority and findings of this RCT, but questions the diagnosis of the women in the control group. Wessely asserts that the women scoring high for anxiety and depression were merely showing signs of 'the post natal blues' which, by his definition, are neither abnormal nor pathological. This study, although appearing to endorse the role of the midwife post natally, actually raises more questions than it answers about both research methods and new mothers' mental health.

At home after the birth

The changes in the continuing provision of support throughout childbearing have been shown to carry benefits post natally as well as at other times (Flint *et al.*, 1989; Oakley, 1992b). But since the publication of the disconcerting findings of an important survey of women's post natal health (MacArthur *et al.*, 1991) many aspects of the care of the new mother have been subjected to scrutiny. The 'routine' post natal care at home is particularly vulnerable to scrutiny and, possibly, amendment (MacArthur, 1999). One aspect of routine supportive post natal care which has been scrutinised and found wanting is home visiting by the midwife. This longstanding system of visiting aims to maintain regular contact with the new mother. In this way the psychological well-being of the mother, which is one crucial aspect of care after the birth, is thought to be enhanced (Garcia *et al.*, 1994).

In spite of these good intentions the research by Marsh and Sargent (1991) indicated the limited significance of the provision of support to the community midwife. These researchers collected data from 24 community midwives over a two week period. They were able to identify the major factors which influenced the duration of the midwife's visit to the woman's home. The data clearly show the likelihood that physical aspects of care, such as examination of the woman and/or baby or the phenylketonuria test, are the most likely aspects to cause the visit to be extended.

Thus, these essentially physical tasks have been suggested as being more important to the midwife than to the woman. This is a sorry reflection on the ability of the midwife to identify and respond to the woman's needs. This conclusion is endorsed by the finding that the duration of the midwife's visit was not affected by the existence of psychosocial problems which might be resolved by supportive intervention. Neither was the duration of visits influenced by the absence of a supportive partner or other family members or friends. The researchers generously assume that the midwife's ability to offer support where it is needed is constrained by her workload. In spite of this, the point is clearly made that an opportunity to make a difference to the woman's experience is being ignored in favour of physical interventions which verge on the routine.

The reference by Marsh and Sargent to constraints on the midwife's time is reinforced by the study by Garcia and colleagues (1994). This study suggests that, although post natal visiting is being used more selectively, the basis of that selection is uncertain. Considerable variation was identified in visiting policies between the 170 English health districts which responded. The researchers argue that the woman's needs should be articulated more explicitly as the basis for deciding who is visited. The suggestion that the woman's need for support may still not be the basis of the midwife's decision about visiting, emerges in a more recent ethnographic study (Hamilton, 1998).

The relationship between the practice of selective visiting and the provision of support may be found in a survey by Poole (1999). Since one of the aims of psychosocial support is the encouragement of self-esteem and confidence (see Chapter 1), Poole's study of anxiety has the potential to define the extent to which support was lacking. Of the 78 questionnaires which were distributed to a variety of new mothers, 46 were returned and were able to be used for analysis. This survey, however, suggests that less frequent visiting by the midwife in the early days is not associated with any difference in the mother's level of anxiety. The meaning of this finding is not entirely clear, as it may mean that the midwife's visits are of no benefit. Disconcertingly, higher levels of anxiety were identified on the days of the midwife's visit than on other days. Whether this means that the midwife's home visits are actually counterproductive in terms of providing social support is difficult to judge.

Conclusion

In this chapter I have attempted to assess whether and to what extent midwifery care provides the support which meets the woman's needs throughout her childbearing experience. In order to answer this question, I have examined some of the multitude of research reports which have studied the effectiveness of midwifery care.

The research suggests that midwifery care and its organisation are undergoing a series of important developments. These have focused around the document usually referred to as *Changing Childbirth* (1993). Its recommendations held out immense promise to women and to midwives of a new order of organisation of maternity care. This promise comprised meeting the needs and aspirations of all who benefited from or provided maternity, and particularly midwifery, care. The potential for woman-centred care with the midwife as the lead professional acted as a spur to midwives to introduce and evaluate a large number of modifications in their traditional practice. Having only been tested by the passage of time, that traditional practice had been found wanting.

In her analysis of the contemporary developments in midwifery, Rothwell (1996) considers the recent recommendations from the point of view of the mother, of the administrator and of the obstetrician. Rothwell concludes that cognisance has been taken of the views of all those involved with the exception of the midwife. Her lack of a political voice has meant that the midwife has permitted her own, and inevitably her client the woman's, needs to be 'pushed hither and thither' (Rothwell, 1996: 292) by whichever authority group is most powerful at the time. To Rothwell this power is held by those who control the financing of the maternity services.

Lewis (1996) also analyses these recent developments, drawing similar conclusions to those of Rothwell. While not actually espousing conspiracy theory, Lewis reiterates Rothwell's perception that the midwife's dedication has been abused by policy makers who control the maternity purse-strings. He states that:

> 'midwives, and midwifery managers in particular, have been set up to fail due to lack of financial support, over-commitment by midwives and lack of commitment by policy makers'.

Thus, I have been suggesting that the midwife may have been manipulated in order to raise the expectations of both care providers and care recipients. The short term financial implications of these developments, however, have prevented their long term implementation. This is also the conclusion reached by Roberts (1996), whose economic interpretation of the benefits of choice regrets the short-termism of a generation of policy makers. She reminds us that the concept of choice was promised not only in the *Changing Childbirth* report, but also in *Working for Patients* (DoH, 1989). Despite this, it is a promise which no longer rings true. The suspicion is that this package may have represented a political carrot which is no longer needed. Thus, for reasons which may be other than related to maternal-child health, innovative midwifery schemes have not been permitted to demonstrate their value, and for a genuine evaluation of their effectiveness, the jury may still be out.

Chapter 5
Support in labour

I examine, in this chapter, the research which has been undertaken to assess the benefits or otherwise of the supportive presence of a labour companion. It has been suggested that the woman's companions form a crucial component of her environment when she is in labour and that this total environment is likely to affect her experience of labour and birth (Hodnett & Osborn, 1989b: 289; Mander, 1998: 139). In the UK the setting in which labour happens changed following the introduction of the National Health Service (NHS) in 1948. Thus, a cascade of changes in the birth environment were initiated by the advent of the NHS. These included the hospitalisation of birth and fundamental changes in the role of the midwife (Robinson, 1990). For these reasons the focus of this chapter is on the supportive nature of the total labour environment. This term is being interpreted broadly here so as to encompass *all* aspects of the woman's surroundings.

The effects of some of the changes in this total labour environment, summarised as 'routines', were the focus of a study by Garcia and Garforth (1989). This study comprised a postal survey of all the consultant maternity units in England. The 93% response rate ($n = 220$) permitted a comprehensive picture of how the respondents (directors of midwifery services) perceived the policies in operation in the labour and delivery services for which they were responsible. As well as what might be termed 'obstetric' policies, such as the use of electronic fetal monitoring, the researchers sought information on the 'comfort and well-being' of the woman in labour. This section included questions about the woman's companions in labour and during the birth. Only 40% of the responding units were able to report that the woman's partner was *never* excluded. The remaining 60% of units could ask him to leave for certain procedures, if a general anaesthetic was administered, if she was moved into the operating theatre or, disconcertingly, 'at the doctor's discretion' (Garcia & Garforth, 1989: 157). The majority of units permitted only one companion to be present. The remainder (31.8%, $n = 70$) did allow another adult companion to remain with the woman in addition to her partner.

It is helpful to bear in mind this, albeit dated, picture of labour care in the UK while considering the research into labour support, because it is necessary to take account of the total environment or context in which each research project was undertaken, including crucially the presence or absence of labour companions.

Understanding this total environment should facilitate an assessment of the implications of the various interventions.

In order to describe the developments in support in labour, I draw on the research literature. While accepting that research may not always present an accurate reflection of the care provided, this literature does demonstrate the wide variation in the standards of care. It also demonstrates wide variations in attitudes towards that care. Thus, it may be that these variations approximate to reality. I address first some important research related issues and then move on to critically analyse the studies.

Research related issues

I attempted to define the meaning of the term 'support' in the first chapter of this book. While this definition is broadly applicable to the events of labour, the context in which the support is provided is clearly more challenging than at other times. The challenges originate primarily in the woman's labour, but the other people and the built environment may also contribute.

In relying on the research literature to assess the effectiveness of social support in labour, it is necessary to recognise the problems of undertaking research in this area. In the context of one particular supportive intervention, Klein (1997) alerts the reader to the likelihood of confounding effects in the research site. It is necessary to bear in mind the close-knit working environment for staff in a setting where women with differing levels of risk are in labour. Klein refers to the 'contamination' of the care of women in uncomplicated labour in such a setting. Because of the human needs of staff, there is little possibility of reducing contact by segregating staff offering the intervention to 'low risk' mothers, from the other staff. Although Klein does not actually mention it, the contamination may operate in both directions. This possibility would serve to further reduce differences between the intervention group and the controls.

The problems of researching support led Oakley (1992c) to question the effect on the supporter and her behaviour if she is being observed. Clearly, the Hawthorne effect, an alteration in behaviour associated with being the subject of research, may operate. This may benefit the individual women, as it is assumed that behaviour improves, but not the data which are collected.

The timing of the collection of the data may be an equally confounding variable in some of the studies to which I refer below. Unsurprisingly and for two main reasons, many researchers collected data while the woman remained in the maternity unit. The first reason relates to the quantitative nature of many of the studies. Due to the large numbers involved, making home visits for data collection would be both inconvenient and expensive. Second, because of the challenging nature of new motherhood the completion of a research instrument is not a priority for the woman, so a 'captive population' is likely to benefit response rates. Following on from this, it is necessary to question whether still being in the maternity unit is likely to have affected the women's responses and in which direction.

The research

In order to critically analyse the research, I use a theoretical framework consisting of the training or professional education of the personnel involved. This aspect was chosen because it is mentioned in all the studies; this is compared with factors such as personal childbearing experience which, although likely to be relevant, are mentioned less consistently. My analysis begins with the situation with which I personally am best acquainted. This situation involves midwives, who are often previously or additionally qualified as nurses, as in the UK. My account then moves through less well-trained care providers, reaching, eventually, the lay woman with no formal training. Although these categories may initially appear quite discrete, there are occasions where the boundaries become blurred, perhaps due to research protocols, to the local availability of staff or to other factors.

The midwife and the nurse-midwife

In spite of the many differences between midwives and their practice in different countries (Mander, 1995, 1997), it is convenient here to regard them as one occupational group. Although this grouping may be superficial, it is supported by the potential of all midwives to work in a variety of settings which correspond with the woman's childbearing cycle. This factor is important when compared with nurses in maternity, whose role appears more tightly circumscribed.

Among the features of labour which make it such an important experience to the woman are the unknowns and unknowables that it brings. These uncertainties make it difficult for the woman to prepare herself and for her attendants to help her to prepare. In spite of the uncertainties, or perhaps because of them, the woman is likely to develop certain expectations which relate to her own functioning and that of her partner and to the behaviour of the staff attending her. By tapping into the woman's expectations, researchers have been able to gain insights into the woman's reactions to her experience of labour.

These expectations emerged in an Ontario study completed prior to midwifery licensing (Soderstrom *et al.*, 1990). A postal questionnaire was used to survey all women giving birth in a two month period ($n = 1929$). The topic, midwifery practice, mattered sufficiently to the women to generate a response rate of 68.4%. The questionnaire sought information on which professional the woman would prefer to provide certain services during her childbearing cycle. The woman could choose between midwife, general practitioner, obstetrician, nurse or childbirth educator. The findings showed that the support expected from the midwife was particularly important to the women. The midwife was preferred to the physician, the obstetrician and the nurse on most of the more supportive services such as education and counselling. This did not apply to the prescription of medicines. Interestingly, though, the services of the nurse were preferred by 62.5% of women to provide support in labour. This is compared with the 50% of women who would have liked midwifery care in labour (the categories do not appear to have been mutually exclusive).

Only 3% of Soderstrom *et al.*'s respondents had experienced the then alegal midwifery care. The responses suggested that 60% of women would seek it at some point. This study served to fuel the impetus for change in Canadian maternity services which soon followed. The findings do suggest, though, that Canadian women initially had difficulty understanding the comprehensive role of the midwife, accustomed as they were to a highly fragmented form of maternity care. This difficulty may have been aggravated by the acrimonious debate between Canadian nurses and midwives about the breadth of the tasks which each would undertake, due to some midwives being reluctant to accept 'nursing' duties.

The high expectations of Soderstrom *et al.*'s Canadian sample are in some ways comparable with those identified by Spiby and colleagues in England (1999). These researchers undertook a within-subjects study ($n = 156$, response rate 87%) which examined the midwife's support for the woman's use of the coping strategies she had learned during pregnancy. Prior to labour the women confidently expected the midwife to prompt and encourage the use of coping strategies (95% and 97% respectively). Fewer women expected the midwife to actually demonstrate it (77%). These researchers found that the reality fell seriously short of the women's expectations. Coping strategies were likely to be encouraged (52%), but demonstrations were only available to 19% of the women. The birth companion was found to be far more likely to meet the woman's expectations, and even occasionally to exceed them. In terms of how these findings reflect on the support offered by the midwife, the researchers suggest that the midwife is reluctant to intervene by giving informational support when the woman and her birth partner appear to be working well together. This, at first glance, appears to be a sorry reflection on the midwife's use of her supportive skills. An alternative explanation is the possibility of a mismatch between what women are taught in childbirth education classes and the model adopted by the midwife. If the woman had been taught to expect directed pushing, or the 'rugby scrum approach' (Thomson, 1993), she might have been disappointed at being encouraged to 'follow her body' (Sleutel, 2000).

The comparison which Spiby and colleagues (1999) were able to make between the woman's expectation of support and her perception of the reality may reflect disparagingly on the midwife's skills. A very different picture of a similar situation is presented by Holroyd and colleagues (1997). Set among the ethnic Chinese women of Hong Kong, this study sought to assess the extent to which the midwife's care in labour was perceived as supportive. The instrument which was used was the Bryanton Adaptation of Nursing Support in Labour Questionnaire

(BANSILQ) (Bryanton *et al.*, 1994). The first part of the instrument comprised a five-point Likert scale, which assessed nursing support behaviours to meet informational, tangible and emotional needs. The second section collected sociodemographic data. The researchers recruited 30 primigravid women to provide a non-random purposive sample. The questionnaire was completed in the post natal ward. The women indicated that their informational and emotional support needs had been met and this was valued more highly than the less important tangible support.

While Holroyd and colleagues admit the limitations of this study, they emphasise its importance in terms of recognising the environment in which labour occurred. This applies partly to the absence of any partner support for the women, as his presence is culturally unacceptable. It applies also to the midwife's ability to enhance the woman's self-esteem, which the authors maintain is significant in view of Chinese women's traditionally subservient role (Holroyd, 1997: 69). The effective emotional support was also an achievement because of the Chinese tendency to 'suppress feelings' (Holroyd, 1997: 69). In spite of these recognisably supportive behaviours, the midwife was able to meet the Chinese women's need to keep a respectful distance and to avoid touching and eye contact; these are considered both impolite and offensive (Holroyd, 1997: 71). Thus, this small study shows how midwives are able to create a culturally acceptable supportive environment in labour.

Whereas the instrument used in the Hong Kong study assessed the woman's informational, tangible and emotional needs, the questionnaire in a Finnish study focused on affirmation, affect and aid (Tarkka & Paunonen, 1996). Two hundred volunteers were recruited over three weeks from women giving birth in one maternity unit. The sample was well-educated, usually accompanied by a partner, and had attended childbirth education. The structured questionnaires were completed in the post natal ward, giving a response rate of 80%. The support by the midwife in labour was perceived as significantly (p = 0.001) more beneficial in the affective domain than for affirmation. The researchers found that first time mothers receive more support in terms of aid and affect and that younger mothers are given more aid. In general terms 85% of the women reported that the labour and birth had been a positive experience. The midwife's presence, encouragement and individual care were felt to have contributed to the experience. The midwife was appreciated, to the extent that the presence of the significant other was regarded as less important than that of the professional.

'Trusting the staff' by the woman was identified as a form of support in a study by Niven (1994). This trust emerged in the women who felt that the (midwifery) staff controlled the total environment and were happy with this. It would appear that Niven's 'trust' corresponds with the woman's perception of being supported. Niven found that 'trust' was associated with significantly lower levels of pain on seven assessments. The differences in pain perception between the trusting or supported women and the others (those who did not consider the staff to be in control or those who thought the staff were in control but were unhappy about it) were also highly significant. There were also positive correlations between 'trusting the staff', effective analgesic medication, effective non-pharmacological pain control and attendance for childbirth education. Niven suggests that childbirth education encourages positive relationships between the midwife and the woman. This may be associated with earlier non-threatening encounters with, albeit different, midwives prior to the stress of labour inhibiting new impressions. The women who trusted the staff were more likely to employ a range of effective coping strategies. Niven argues that these strategies, such as relaxation, are more easily attempted and utilised successfully within a trusting, supportive environment.

A phenomenological study in Sweden also identified that a trusting, supportive environment for the labour was appreciated by the woman (Lundgren & Dahlberg, 1998). The researchers were seeking to describe the experience of labour pain. Nine women, none of whom had used either opioids or epidural analgesia, agreed to participate following an uncomplicated birth. The findings were profound, relating to the meaning of life rather than just the labour. Two of the four major themes which emerged featured trust, in the woman herself and her body, and in the midwife and the partner. These women spoke of withdrawing during labour using terms such as 'You go into yourself' (Lundgren & Dahlberg, 1998: 107). The researchers conclude that coping ability is innate in a woman's body. They warn, however, that it is necessary for the midwife to maintain a supportive environment to allow the woman to interpret her body's signals. If the midwife fails in this, the woman's trust in the midwife, the partner and the environment is likely to be diminished by the intrusion of outside influences.

The ability of the midwife to engender a supportive environment appears to matter to the childbearing woman. Further, this environment may assume a variety of forms. One of these manifested itself in a study which clearly demonstrated the cultural impact of certain potentially supportive behaviours, such as the use of touch (Holroyd *et al.*, 1997). An American researcher investigated the use of touch in labour among 30 women whose labour was attended by a nurse-midwife (Birch, 1986). The therapeutic value of touch was investigated using structured interviews undertaken in the post natal ward. All of the women had experienced touch during labour and a marginally smaller proportion had found touch very helpful in coping with labour (97%). Only one woman was neutral in her response to touch. Although clearly limited in its value, Birch's study informs a topic which will emerge as increasingly significant as this chapter and the next examine the provision of support in labour.

There is concern about the effects on a research project of caring for women experiencing uncomplicated birth in the same clinical area as 'high risk' women (Klein, 1997, see above). Also contemplating the likelihood of 'contamination', Hundley and colleagues (1994) sought to assess whether midwife-managed births (in a midwife-managed delivery unit or MMDU) could be offered in close proximity to a consultant-led labour area. The researchers recognised that the choice of home birth is currently less frequently offered and aimed to make up for this by providing safe care in a 'homely environment' (Hundley *et al.*, 1994: 1400). The Aberdeen MMDU was separate, but only approximately 20 m from the main labour ward. Minimal technology and limited intervention in labour were utilised and there was no input from medical staff. The staffing of the MMDU was from the same pool of midwives as the labour ward. Working within strict protocols, of the 3451 eligible women 2844 (82.4%) were recruited and randomised at booking for either MMDU care in labour or standard care. To allow for the likelihood of transfers two women were randomised to MMDU care for every one that was randomised to labour ward care. Data were collected by questionnaires to the staff and to the women and by 400 random interviews. In spite of a high transfer rate, midwifery care was shown to be safe and effective. The data may allow an assessment of the effectiveness of the support offered by MMDU midwives by focusing on the pain control methods. Natural methods and TENS (transcutaneous electrical nerve stimulation) were significantly more likely (p = 0.001) to be used in the MMDU and epidural analgesia was significantly less likely to be used by these women (p = 0.05).

The findings presented by Rennie and colleagues (1998) present a somewhat different impression of the support offered by the MMDU. On the basis of the women's questionnaires and interviews, these findings suggest that the women changed their minds about who is important at the birth. The authors make no claims that women's changed views reflect on their care, but I have to question whether women's views could not be seriously affected by an experience like giving birth. Rennie and colleagues show that with the birth the woman's partner or other birth companion becomes significantly (p = 0.0003) more important to her. On the other hand, even the known midwife becomes significantly (p = 0.0010) less important. Although they had intended to, these researchers were unable to evaluate the importance of the constant attendance of a midwife. This was because the researchers altered the question in the post natal questionnaire due to 'the women valuing their option of choice more highly' (Rennie *et al.*, 1998: 435).

In the same way as Soderstrom and colleagues (1990, above) sought data relating to the forthcoming legalisation of midwifery in Canada, Kaufman and McDonald (1988) assessed the differences between midwife and physician care in labour. This retrospective study involved the review of the charts of 79 women attended by a midwife and 373 women attended by a physician. The outcomes were only those which had already been measured or counted, so no assessment of 'soft' variables such as support was included. In spite of this these findings provide a useful impression of the nature of maternity care in Canada before the midwifery legislation. Examples include the significantly (p = 0.034) increased likelihood of a woman attended by a midwife sustaining a perineal laceration, or being significantly (p = 0.016) less likely to use epidural analgesia. The findings show the midwife's less interventive approach, with significantly (p = 0.026) less (and later) use of amniotomy and significantly (p = 0.002) more use of TENS. This comparison is useful because it shows the contrast in certain areas of practice which may reflect the support offered by midwifery care as opposed to standard care. This standard medicalised care, usually involving labour and delivery room (LDR) nurses, constitutes the baseline from which later recommendations for support have been made throughout north America. This standard care, incorporating nursing support, and the associated recommendations are examined in the next section.

The nurse

In order to examine the extent to which the nurse is able to provide support to the woman in labour, it is necessary to consider the system of health care within which she practises. In Chapter 2 I focused on examples of relevant health systems and considered the maternity related issues. It is sufficient to mention here that if the nurse per se contributes systematically and significantly to maternity care, it is as an extension of the medicalised organisation of care. For this reason the nurse's support in labour assumes a crucially different significance from that provided by the midwife. When considering nursing support the medicalised environment in which that childbirth happens needs to be taken into account to better understand the woman's need for support.

A Canadian study undertaken by Shields, even though it was published in 1978, demonstrates some important issues relating to the support provided by nurses during labour. The new mothers ($n = 80$) were asked about nurses' activities and what had been most helpful and least helpful. The structured interviews were based on a questionnaire, which also asked about numbers of nurses and companions. The woman's care was categorised as physical only, supportive only, medication only or any combination. Her satisfaction was rated on a five-point scale. The results showed that 32% of the women ($n = 25$) reported physical care only, and 34% ($n = 27$) reported supportive and physical care. A majority of the women ($n = 45$, 56%) stated that supportive care was the most helpful. The presence of the nurse was the most frequently mentioned aspect of supportive care by 25% of the women ($n = 20$). The data collection for this study may be criticised on the grounds that the interviews were by 16 nursing students who were caring for the women in the maternity unit within four days of the birth. Additionally, the data collection instrument appears quite inflexible.

The study by Shields provides useful insights into the environment, the care provided and the women's views about them. The women were largely alone in labour as partners/fathers were not ordinarily present. While in labour 45 women (56%) were 'visited' and this was usually by their partner, but there is no indication of how long the visitor stayed. The fact that one woman 'had her mother and sister with her' (Shields, 1978: 545), suggests that these companions were able to stay throughout the labour, but that this was unusual. An attempt was made to assess the importance of visitors. Shields found that visitors made no significant difference to the women's nursing needs. The women's views about the importance of their visitors was variable, with six women (7.5%) stating that they preferred to be alone in labour. Shields recommends that the nurse should be able to recognise the woman's 'need/non-need' for her presence as this is crucial to her satisfaction with her care. This recommendation appears to suggest that the women did not seek company continuously, although it is necessary to question whether this is a reflection of the reality of the care provided.

The impression which this study leaves is of normal labour being any birthing experience not involving a caesarean or one or more of three serious complications. 'Monitoring' does not appear to have been routine in Canada then, but perineal shaves and enemas were and the reference to bedpans suggests that the woman was confined to bed. The crucial role of support is shown in Shields' conclusion that the supportiveness of care was what differentiated satisfaction with care from dissatisfaction. The nurse's helpful contribution is reflected in the fact that the time spent with the woman is predictive of her satisfaction with her care. Thus, it appears that a less than supportive environment may have been ameliorated by nursing interventions.

Certain important issues are raised by a more recent study which was undertaken in the USA by Corbett and Callister (2000). In order to emphasise the importance of support in labour, these researchers record the following rather negative observation:

> 'Few human experiences approach the intensity of emotions, stress, anxiety, pain and exertion that can occur during labour and birth.'
>
> (Corbett & Callister, 2000: 71)

The highly appropriate theoretical framework which was used for this study comprised social support as an environmental coping resource. This study bears some resemblance to the one undertaken by Holroyd and colleagues (1997) (see earlier section 'The midwife and the nurse-midwife') in that, first, support was categorised as emotional, informational and tangible and second, the BANSILQ was the data collection instrument. Corbett and Callister, with due regard to the important role of nurse, sought to identify the nursing behaviours that are helpful to the woman in labour. The five-point Likert scale which was used showed a high level of satisfaction among the women with the emotional support provided. This is apparent in that 16 out of the 25 behaviours (64%) produced a mean score of greater than 4.00, indicating that they were definitely helpful. The researchers were also able to conclude that emotional support was more highly valued than tangible or informational support.

The research site for this study provides useful insights and raises important issues relating to care. The setting was a level three birthing unit in a tertiary care medical centre in which there were 4000 births per annum. The majority of births took place in a birthing room. The staffing is described as '1:1 or 1:2 in active labour' which, hopefully, means that each actively labouring woman was attended by two nurses. The data were collected while the woman was in the recovery room or in the mother-baby unit and the 88 women who were approached gave a 100% return rate. This relatively affluent sample were able to choose their pain control method and 93% chose epidural analgesia during their labour. The remaining 7% are described as having an unmedicated labour.

Corbett and Callister (2000) state that they interpret the data as showing that the woman's need for emotional support was validated by this study, irrespective of the method of pain control employed. They do admit, however, that more research is necessary in this area. This study clearly raises the question of whether there is any difference in the quality or the intensity of support needed for a woman with an effective system of epidural analgesia in progress. It may be assumed that a large component of support in labour serves to assist the woman's ability to work with, to accept or to cope with the pain she experiences. The other anxieties may have been assumed to be less burdensome in comparison. The work of Morgan *et al.* (1982) found that epidural analgesia, although effective in controlling labour pain, did not make the woman more satisfied with her birth experience. Morgan's study, though, involved the use of epidural analgesia as a 'last resort', when other methods of pain control had been found wanting. In the Corbett and Callister (2000) study, however, epidural analgesia appears to have been the method of choice. One of the multitude of questions which this study does not answer relates to the extent to which labour was in any way challenging for these women and, thus, the value of their support.

In the research literature on support in labour (Hodnett & Osborn, 1989a; Keirse *et al.*, 1989; Hofmeyr & Nikodem, 1994) the Dublin 'experience' invariably features prominently (O'Driscoll *et al.*, 1993). These obstetricians maintain that the support which is provided for the woman in labour is crucial to the success of their protocol. This success is usually assessed, at least in the North American literature, by the unusually low caesarean rate in first time mothers. In the third edition of their 'manual', O'Driscoll (1993: 9) and his colleagues report a caesarean rate of 5% among primigravid women. Later in the same volume the rate is shown to have risen to 8.5% by 1992 (O'Driscoll, 1993: 191). O'Regan (1998: 6) maintains that this low, but apparently rising, caesarean rate is the major reason for the North American interest in the Dublin regime. She argues that these rates have proved the unique selling point of active management of labour to North Americans, due to their concerns about their 'escalating' caesarean rates. While O'Regan does not explicitly link this North American interest with the subsequent epidemic of labour support research by physicians there, the connection is clear. O'Regan does, however, draw attention to the less well publicised, high, perinatal mortality rates and the limited relevance of the Dublin protocol to cultures featuring smaller families.

The underlying rationale for the Dublin system of support is found in their belief in the causative relationship between technical surveillance/intervention and the woman's feelings of isolation. The woman closing her eyes is held to be of profound significance, indicating, it is maintained, a tendency to introspection, the onset of panic and 'the first step along the road to total disintegration' (O'Driscoll *et al.*, 1993: 93). The ultimate outcome of such panic is said to threaten marital harmony and the mother–child relationship. The woman is said, by these obstetricians, to be guaranteed continuous personal attention throughout her labour. The allocation of 'one nurse to one patient' is said to facilitate this level of attention (O'Driscoll, 1993: 93). The mere physical presence of the companion, however, is not considered enough. The companion is required to provide the emotional support needed, and this is distinct from clinical activities. Part of the nurse's responsibility, and a clear indicator of the submissive role of the woman, is to 'ensure the mother genuinely understands the purpose of each medical procedure' (O'Driscoll, 1993: 94) and is kept informed. The Dublin National Maternity Hospital's guarantee of 'a personal nurse through the whole of labour' is only feasible if the duration of labour is limited. In this way the support system and the active, some might say aggressive, management of labour are seen to be interdependent.

The support which is provided comprises personal care by one staff member for one woman each day. It is given by the nurse sitting in a face-to-face posture with direct eye contact and without others being present. The staff member is not permitted to leave the woman in labour. If the woman chooses to walk the two walk together. In order to provide distraction, conversation may be on any subject. At all costs eye closing must be prevented.

While some may consider that this harsh regime may be justified by the measurable outcomes, such as short duration of labour (Anderson, 2000) and low caesarean rates (O'Driscoll *et al.*, 1993: 191, 205), this is questionable. The inconsistencies of the protocol become apparent with close scrutiny.

First, the research basis of this regime is negligible to the point of absence. Keirse (1993), in his heretical lampoon of the Dublin regime, makes this observation in relation to myometrial inefficiency. This criticism may also be applied to the general application of this form of support, to the 'eye closing' veto and the eye contact, which actually contradict research (Lundgren & Dahlberg, 1998; Holroyd *et al.*, 1997). It is clear that, as observed by Keirse, far from being based on research and even less on evidence this regime is actually 'based on beliefs and assumptions' (Keirse, 1993: 160).

The second inconsistency may be found in the provider of the support, which is an example of the 'blurring' to which I referred earlier in this chapter. Frequently this person is referred to as a 'nurse', although O'Driscoll and colleagues (1993: 17, 100) regard the terms 'nurse' and 'midwife' and 'student midwife' as 'interchangeable because all are general trained'. This lack of distinction may be disconcerting, especially for those concerned with midwifery education. The gender of the supporter is frequently emphasised: 'In our experience young, properly motivated girls perform this task with remarkable success' (O'Driscoll, 1993: 102). In the interests of medical education, however, medical students of the male gender appear to be equally well-qualified to offer this quintessentially feminine form of support in labour. The conditions under which the medical student functions are strictly enforced: 'He is given to understand that the commitment to a woman in labour must be absolute' (O'Driscoll & Meagher, 1986: 85).

Third, regardless of their discipline or level of education, the support person appears to have considerable responsibility. This is because the care of the woman in labour, both in terms of support and clinical expertise, is by this one person alone. If the observations of the vital signs are actually only made as infrequently as at 'intervals of two hours' (O'Driscoll *et al.*, 1993: 93) this should leave the support person with time to concentrate on supporting.

In summary, the Dublin regime presents a picture of a form of management of labour which verges on the 'military efficiency' to which the authors refer (O'Drisoll & Meagher, 1986: 89). It is this very efficiency which, we are told, permits the much admired system of support. The environment of care, though, is characterised by the dominance of the partograph to determine the timing and extent of interventions to augment labour. This labour environment has been appropriately described as 'neo-Taylorist ' after 'Speedy Taylor', who was one of the twentieth century's less humane occupational psychologists (Mason, 2000: 247). It is necessary to consider whether the labour ward environment in Dublin's National Maternity Hospital is only rendered tolerable (if it is) by the presence of the support person.

The question that remains relates to the low caesarean rate for first time mothers and to its attribution, if it is not to the system of support in labour. An explanation may be found in O'Driscoll *et al.* (1993: 207, Table 9). This table indicates the stage of labour at which women are admitted to the National Maternity Hospital. It shows that 5% of primigravidae have achieved full dilatation of the cervix prior to admission to the maternity unit. These figures are not normally recorded, but in over 30 years as a midwife I am unable to recall such a situation in uncomplicated childbirth. It becomes necessary to question whether the low caesarean rate is due to this artefact rather than to the support system. This leads in turn to the question of why the rate of primigravid full dilatation on admission is so high. There may, after all, be some truth to the infamous anecdote of women sitting outside the National Maternity Hospital Dublin in labour on a park bench, thus delaying admission and inevitable intervention and, coincidentally, avoiding caesarean.

It is becoming clear that the environment in which the woman labours comprises a range of aspects which may be more or less conducive to, or requiring of, support. It may be that the accounts mentioned already indicate that a more medicalised birth experience carries with it, by way of compensation, the requirement for more supportive care. A case study of a relatively highly medicalised and interventive labour/delivery unit focused on the implications of the environment in the form of the relationships between nursing and medical personnel (Sleutel, 2000). This researcher provides minimal detail about the research site. The reader is informed that it is modern, in Texas and with about 1000 births per annum. The practice of the nursing and medical staff is simply described as being 'typical for the region' (Sleutel, 2000: 39). The data collection comprised observation and interviews with one informant, which was followed by qualitative data analysis to create a case study. This study discusses support in terms of emotional support, information/advice, physical support, partner support and advocacy. Of particular importance was the presence of the nurse in the form of 'just being there'. Additionally a positive attitude manifested itself in 'lots of encouragement' and 'talking it up'; the latter refers to putting a positive 'spin' on any aspect of labour. Thus, these forms of emotional support were crucial, whereas physically supportive care was of least significance.

In the relationship between the nursing and medical personnel, according to Sleutel, caesareans appear to be pivotal. 'Carrie', the name given to the nurse who is the subject of the case study, is anxious to prevent caesareans and to facilitate each mother's 'natural' birth. The physician's priority, however, appears to be his 'golf game' (Sleutel, 2000: 40). Thus, conflict emerges between obeying the physician's instructions and meeting the woman's needs. This conflict appears to be aggravated by the likelihood of substandard medical care. Not surprisingly, nurse-physician conflict is only narrowly avoided. Credit for avoiding open conflict appears to be due to the nurse, whose strategies are reminiscent of those identified in midwives working in a labour ward by Walker (1976) and by the well-known recommendation of 'doing good by stealth'. Although not explicitly mentioned by Sleutel, the question that this case study raises relates to the nurse's accountability. The nurse's legal situation is not explained, but her ethical duty is abundantly plain. The anxiety remains, however, that the woman's welfare may be threatened to some extent by the nurse's loyalty to her physician colleagues.

Through the work of Sleutel another aspect of the labour environment begins to emerge: the loyalty of the person who provides support and/or care. For Sleutel's 'Carrie', her loyalty appeared to be split or at least shared between the woman in labour and the physician. Sagady (1997) moves this debate forward by suggesting that the nurse's clinical responsibility and loyalty renders ineffective her support for the woman in labour. According to this writer, who is a director of the Association of Labor Assistants and Childbirth Educators, those who also carry clinical duties are unable to offer support simultaneously. Unsurprisingly, Sagady recommends the additional attendance of a labour support provider, who is responsible only to the woman and the family. The professional labour support provider is described as preferable to nurses, because of having no clinical duties, and to lay support providers, due to her greater knowledge.

The issue of the support person's loyalty is further explored by Hodnett (1997) from a North American perspective. She maintains that nurses are less than acceptable as supporters because, like other employees, they are constrained by hospital policies. On this basis Hodnett (1997: 78) 'doubts that hospital employees can be effective providers of labour support'. Hodnett discusses how nurses, in their roles as employees, are formally constrained by the policies of their employing organisation. She also refers to the informal or social role of the nurse within the labour/delivery environment. In the setting that she describes there exists a norm of spending more time in social interaction with nurse colleagues, as opposed to spending time with the woman in labour. Hodnett appears to be sympathetic to the individual nurse's need to conform to the informal social organisation of the area in which she is employed. After arguing that who supports is less significant than the fact that support is provided, Hodnett (1997: 80) goes on to advocate that support is best provided by a woman 'with no prior social bond'. This latter recommendation appears to contradict the recommendations for continuity and named carer which have recently become fundamental aims of UK maternity care, as discussed in Chapter 4. That the standard of nursing care provided for the woman in labour is as low as Hodnett indicates may surprise some who read her work. It is crucially important to bear Hodnett's observations in mind when reading other work by this prolific and authoritative writer. It is now appropriate to scrutinise the research basis of these observations about the labour and delivery environment.

A study of the effectiveness of the nurse's support in labour, undertaken in Montreal, provides some helpful insights into the Canadian labour environment (Gagnon *et al.*, 1997). These researchers decided to study nurse support simply because of her established presence in the labour/delivery area. This implies a 'convenience sample', rather than the nurse having been shown to be a more effective support person. In Gagnon and colleagues' study the women were randomised only when labour was established. The one-to-one support offered by the nurse to the woman comprised physical comfort measures, emotional support (including reassurance, encouragement, praise and distraction) and instruction on relaxation and coping techniques. The nurse also offered support to the partner. The nurse's constant presence was emphasised to the extent that her 'time out' was strictly limited. Gagnon and colleagues feel confident in concluding that the nurse is the appropriate and effective carer in labour. This conclusion is based on having identified a 'beneficial trend' towards a reduction in the use of oxytocin.

There are, however, a number of serious limitations to Gagnon and colleagues' study. First, the researchers correctly identify that general staff awareness or the 'contamination' mentioned at the beginning of this chapter may have been a problem. The control group may have been better cared for to compensate, thus confounding statistical analyses. Second, due to limited research funds, the recruitment of the intervention nurses proved difficult. This resulted in 563 eligible women not being recruited to the study because no intervention nurse was available. Other aspects of this study further illuminate the nursing care provided in labour. This relates particularly to the period of time before the woman was randomised, that is before she was in established labour. The mean time of this period was five hours, but it allowed time for a number of interactions or interventions which may have influenced the woman's subsequent supportive care. One example which is described is the encouragement or pressure applied to the woman to avail herself of epidural analgesia. As I have described (Mander, 1997) and the authors admit, it is likely that the woman would have been asked on admission and several times thereafter whether this is her chosen method of pain control. The researchers suggest that interventions prior to randomisation may have served to undermine the effectiveness of nurse support and to reduce the significance of the findings.

The poor impression of nursing care in labour which appears to be emerging is further supported by two studies which used work sampling techniques. It may be that the length of time the carer spends in the presence of the labouring woman is not an ideal way of measuring the effectiveness of her provision of a supportive environment. This is because the assumption of work sampling is that the individual member of staff is only able to perform one function at any given time. For example, I would be able while taking a woman's axillary temperature to hold a supportive conversation. In this situation, however, the work sampler would only observe the thermometer and record a clinical activity, without recording the supportive human interaction. This is because work sampling theory requires that the worker's activities are 'mutually exclusive' (McNiven *et al.*, 1992).

In spite of this limitation, McNiven and colleagues (1992) used this technique in an attempt to assess the quality and quantity of support by nurses for women in labour. The research site was the labour and delivery area of a teaching hospital in Toronto. The unit admitted 3600 relatively affluent women per year with, presumably, an equivalent number of births. The staffing of the labour and delivery area, which becomes significant, was sufficient to provide one-to-one nursing care for each woman in established labour. Of particular interest is the unit's 80% epidural rate. Making observations in the daytime only, supportive direct care activities were categorised into four groups: physical comfort, emotional support, instruction and/or information, and advocacy. Additionally the nurse's other work was classified according to other direct care, indirect care and all other activities.

McNiven and colleagues claim that this study shows the limited nursing time spent supporting the woman in labour. While the authors recognise the complexity of providing support in labour, they found that supportive care occupied only 9.9% of the nurse's time. A far larger proportion of the nurse's time was seen to be spent on other forms of direct care, particularly technical tasks, and also on indirect care, such as technical tasks carried out away from the woman's presence. McNiven and colleagues conclude that providing a supportive environment is not a nursing priority and that it tends to be attributed less importance than technical tasks and medically prescribed care. This explanation is related by these researchers to the low status of nursing care in this labour and delivery setting. The lack of continuity of care for the labouring woman is further identified and referred to in terms of 'fragmentation' (McNiven, 1992: 7). This verdict appears to be particularly apposite in the context of this research method and labour environment.

Unlike McNiven and colleagues, Gagnon and Waghorn (1996) undertook their work sampling study on a 24 hour per day and seven day per week basis. As usual, the sampling frame for the work sampling exercise was mutually exclusive and collectively exhaustive. The nurse's work was categorised according to supportive care (physical, emotional, instruction, advocacy), other direct care, indirect care in the room, indirect care outside the room, postpartum care, and time away from the unit. The findings are broadly similar to those of McNiven and colleagues, but more detail of the nurse's activity is provided.

Gagnon and Waghorn found that supportive care was being provided by the nurse for only 6.1% of her time. The nurse spent more of her time with the first time mother (9.2%), but whether or not epidural analgesia was being provided made no difference to the woman's care. In comparison, the indirect care provided outside the room made up 47.6% of the nurse's time, of which 16% involved giving or receiving reports. Twelve per cent of the nurse's time was used in preparing medication and an equal proportion with writing documentation. The time that the nurse spent away from the unit was found to occupy 27.3% of her working time.

Writing that they are 'disturbed' by these findings, Gagnon and Waghorn (1996: 4) suggest that the provision of supportive care is 'too low to be believed'. It is possible, as mentioned at the beginning of this chapter, that the nurses being observed changed their behaviour. This possibility is even more disconcerting as it suggests that their usual care would provide even less time for support. If the definition of support were to be relaxed to include simply the nurse's presence as supportive, then the support time would only be increased to 16.7%. While it may also be possible to construe that even though away from the woman the nurse is 'available' to her, this would not make much difference to the observation that 74.9% of the nurse's time was spent apart from the woman. The possibility of being 'available' clearly cannot apply to the quarter of the nurse's working time spent off the unit.

Gagnon and Waghorn discuss the nurse's perception of her role during labour. She is likely to regard herself as not being needed if the woman's partner is present, if monitoring is in progress or if the woman has an epidural. This self-assessment is not just a sad reflection on nursing skills. Yet again these authors suggest that technical care predominates in this medicalised labour environment, with the emphasis misplaced from supporting the woman to watching the machine. I have suggested that work sampling may not be the best way to record supportive nursing activities. In spite of this criticism, I have to question how the nurse is able to provide care for the woman in labour when she is in her presence for such a small proportion of her working time.

Although published in a midwifery journal produced in the UK, a Canadian study by Beaton and Gupton (1990) investigated, like Soderstrom *et al.* (1990) and Spiby *et al.* (1999) mentioned earlier, the pregnant woman's expectations of the support available to her in labour. This qualitative study is particularly valuable in supporting the two work sampling studies by showing the low expectations that the woman has for the nurse's care during labour and for the supportive environment. The nurse's role is regarded as being merely an adjunct to the physician and as having a monitoring role. The woman's partner or labour coach is generally expected to provide care, support and to meet most of the woman's emotional needs. Only four out of the eleven women informants expected any form of emotional support from the nurse and the majority of women had little idea of the nurse's role: 'I'm not sure what they do'. The researchers regard the women's expectations for the partner as unrealistic and far too high for him to meet. It is necessary to question, though, the origin of these expectations as they are surprisingly similar to the real-life findings of the work sampling studies mentioned. More importantly, however, this study, together with the work sampling studies, demonstrates the unsupportive and over-medicalised context for Hodnett's recommendations for the introduction of changes in the personnel who provide supportive care in labour.

Lay women with training

Having scrutinised the research literature on the support provided by professional carers in labour, the theme which is emerging is the importance of the environment within which the woman labours. The extent to which the midwife or nurse is able to support the woman within a particular context is uncertain. The environment may manifest itself in the lack of humanity of the medicalised or interventionist approaches to care or in the relationships or lack of them between the various actors. In examining the research literature by moving in the direction of less qualified personnel, it is now appropriate to look at the work undertaken on the support provided by lay women who have been trained as labour supporters.

I begin this section by considering the RCT undertaken in a public hospital in Mexico (Langer *et al.*, 1998; Campero *et al.*, 1998). Although I refer to the women who provided support as 'lay women', there is an element of the 'blurring' of boundaries to which I referred earlier. The researchers chose to recruit seven retired nurses in addition to four 'young women' for training as labour supporters. On the basis of what the work sampling studies above have shown of the nurse's care during labour, it is necessary to consider whether the retired nurse's previous training and experience would have affected her functioning as a labour supporter. These 11 women underwent a three week period of training to prepare them to act as what the authors refer to as 'doulas'. These authors define 'doula' as 'a Greek word meaning a woman who accompanies another woman' (Campero *et al.*, 1998: 395).

The training covered practical and theoretical topics. The doula was taught to provide cognitive, physical and emotional support with the intention of enhancing the woman's emotional state during labour. The authors state that this was to be achieved 'simply' through talking, encouraging, soothing, recognising efforts, finding comfortable positions, facilitating relaxation/breathing/pushing, massaging, hand holding, giving bedpans and helping to change clothes. Particularly demanding activities which were expected of the doula after the three week course included 'giving information, explaining medical interventions and answering questions'. The doula was also encouraged to maintain eye contact, the benefits of which have been discussed in this chapter in the context of work by other researchers and writers (Holroyd *et al.*, 1997; O'Driscoll *et al.*, 1993).

The environment of labour featured highly medicalised and interventive practice. The maternity unit was large with 4800 births per annum. Each woman was discharged within 24 hours of the birth. The process of labour was usually viewed as pathological, resulting in a tendency to induce or medically intervene. No partner or other chosen person was allowed to enter the labour ward, leaving the woman effectively 'alone' (Campero *et al.*, 1998: 396). The authors compare this modern labour experience with the woman's 'traditional' care involving a midwife, the family or local women of the community. The context of this study appears to be a society in transition, which results in a serious decline in the support provided in labour. Campero and colleagues emphasise the likelihood of an increase in the woman's anxiety, which results in 'patient compliance' being the norm. The humanity ordinarily shown to the woman in labour was notable by its absence and any comments were likely to aggravate the situation. Information for the woman was also seriously lacking, tending only to be gleaned by eaves-dropping on staff conversations. The woman's emotional needs were not regarded as important.

In this setting first time mothers were recruited and randomised in labour if the cervix was less than 6 cm dilated. This resulted in an intervention group of 360 women and 364 controls. Data which were collected on medical interventions showed no significant difference, but there was some improvement in breast feeding rates. The psychosocial changes, which emerged through the qualitative aspect of the study (Campero *et al.*, 1998), may be more important. The intervention group expressed satisfaction with their functioning in labour, whereas the control group thought that the medical attendants were responsible for the success of the labour and birth. The experiment group found the continuous presence of the doula helpful and that talking to her assisted the woman's coping. Thus, a sense of achievement and having been in control was noted among the experiment group. An external locus of control was more likely to be identified among the control group. The women were particularly appreciative of the doula's explanations of what medical staff and nursing staff had said.

The limited impact of support on medical interventions is due to the strict hospital protocols, according to Langer *et al.* (1998). The psychosocial benefits of the intervention are more easily apparent, in that the doula served to ameliorate an unsupportive, even hostile, labour environment. The example of the doula explaining communication, however, serves to alert the reader to the role of the doula as an intermediary. It may be that her presence served to perpetuate the lack of direct communication, such as when medical personnel speak to the doula rather than directly to the woman. Thus, while the short term benefits of support are clearly apparent, the longer term and underlying problems may not be being addressed.

The RCT by Hodnett and Osborn (1989a, b), like the Mexico study (Campero *et al.*, 1998), features some blurring of the support person's training or professional status. This study was undertaken in Toronto, so the labour environment described in the previous section should also be borne in mind. The environment, however, may have been rendered relatively more supportive by the presence of the partner, as for only one woman was he unable to stay with her. The researchers aimed to assess whether the previous findings on support in labour could be replicated in a more sophisticated setting. Hodnett and Osborn (1989b) argue that the Guatamalan findings are not generalisable to North American birth environments because routine intrapartum practices are very different in the two cultures.

The intervention applied by Hodnett and Osborn comprised the random allocation of the pregnant women to receive either individualised professional support by a familiar monitrice or standard care. The 'monitrices' (Hodnett & Osborn, 1989b) who acted as support persons in labour were eight lay midwives. They were self employed labour coaches, who had been in practice for a year or more and who had cared for at least 20 women during labour. The monitrice was expected to assume a role which was compared with that of the community midwife in the UK. As well as the usual North American care in labour, mentioned earlier, it is also necessary to bear in mind that these monitrices were assuming this role at a time when momentous change in maternity care and the associated powerful feelings prevailed in Canada. Effectively, their position may be comparable with that of Daniel entering the lion's den.

Although 145 women were recruited, the final sample comprised only 49 experiment women and 54 in the control group. In each group all but one were first time mothers. The mother in the experimental group was found to be more likely to have her labour augmented, she was less likely to receive analgesic medication, and she was more likely to sustain an intact perineum. As Campero *et al.* (1998) found, the woman's perception of control over her experience was increased among those in the experimental group. The data tend to support other studies' findings of the low standard of labour and delivery care in North American maternity units (see previous section), such as the lack of physical comfort measures and advocacy support offered by nurses during labour. As usual, the partner is shown to be crucially important to the woman's care, although the women in the experiment group received less information/instruction from their partners. The helpful role of physical touch emerged as being culturally acceptable.

Each of the women in the experimental group met their monitrice during pregnancy. She went to the woman's home when labour was beginning and accompanied the woman into the maternity unit. The monitrice was then required to 'stay with' the couple during labour (Hodnett & Osborn, 1989b: 179). It is unfortunate that 'staying with' the couple is not defined. It is uncertain whether the monitrice was required to be continuously present or whether she was able to take long periods of time out, as was shown to be usual by the work sampling studies. The companionship requirement should have been spelt out, as it has been well-defined in others' work such as that by Gagnon *et al.* (1997). This omission from the account of the supportive environment becomes more important with the greater salience of continuity and the emphasis on the supporter's actual physical presence.

Like Hodnett and Osborn (1989a, b), Kennell and colleagues (1991) sought to assess whether the earlier support studies undertaken in central America were applicable in the supposedly more sophisticated North American setting. This sophistication applied particularly to the 'technologically advanced obstetric units in US hospitals' (Kennell *et al.*, 1991: 2197) where electronic fetal monitoring is described as being routinely used and epidural 'anaesthesia' is widely available. The bottom line becomes clear when these authors reflect on the possibility of reducing the caesarean rate, and the resulting benefits to quality and costs. These reflections resonate strongly with the comments by O'Regan (1998) about the Dublin regime (see previous section).

In Houston, Texas, Kennell and colleagues identified 412 eligible first time mothers in labour. The women were recruited and randomly assigned to a supported group of 212 women or to an observed group of 200 women. By way of a methodological afterthought, a retrospective non-random control group comprising 204 women was later recruited. The intervention comprised the allocation of a doula to the woman in labour. Eleven doulas were recruited, but 82% of the births were attended by one of only four of them. The doulas were aged from 22 to 55 years, were fluent in Spanish and in English and had personal experience of childbearing. These women underwent a three week training, during which they became familiar with normal and abnormal labour, obstetric procedures, hospital policies and a wide variety of supportive techniques.

The doula in Kennell and colleagues' (1991) study was paid from research funds on an hourly basis, which averaged about $200 per woman supported. The doula was not previously known to the woman but she introduced herself by name and explained that she had no expertise in the maternity area other than having given birth herself. The doula told the woman that she would stay at her bedside from admission until the birth, soothing, touching and encouraging (Bulger, 1999). She explained what was happening and what was likely to happen. The doula also acted as an interpreter when necessary. The doula kept a written record of her activities. The women in the observed group experienced the routine hospital care and the observer kept a record of that care. The observer stood in the corner of the room where the woman was in labour wearing a white coat and holding a clipboard. She did not introduce herself, neither did she speak to anyone. She was asked to try to be inconspicuous (Bulger, 1999).

This research was undertaken by Kennell and colleagues (1991) in a public hospital among a low income population of blacks, whites and women of Hispanic origin. The labour and delivery environment for most of the women was a 12 bed ward. This meant that there was insufficient privacy to allow visitors so companions were not routinely present during the labour and the birth. Only brief visits by family were permitted if the labour area was 'not too busy' (Kennell *et al.*, 1991: 2198). It appears that the labour environment lacked continuous support and the only companions were strangers. The standard of care is demonstrated by the information that the woman was bedfast after admission to allow for electronic fetal monitoring, and intravenous infusion and amniotomy were routine. An impression of the labour environment is gained from the finding that the staff interacted with each woman for 21% of the time the woman was in labour. Although this is only a small proportion of her labour, it is more than the 9.2% identified in Montreal (Gagnon & Waghorn, 1996). The restriction on companions resulted in a family member being with the woman for an average of only 4.65% of the duration of her labour.

The supported women were found to experience the shortest labours and to be the least likely to give birth by caesarean or to use epidural analgesia. Comparisons drawn between the doula's support and the partner's support (when given) showed that he touched less and was close less often. That the mere presence of the observer improved the incidence of the major variables suggests the importance of the companionship of another human being.

The background of the women recruited as doulas deserves attention. They all had personal experience of childbearing and underwent what must have been a highly intensive three week training. The doula was not acquainted with the woman. The cultural implications of the intervention, which prominently featured the doula's use of touch, may be variably acceptable in other settings. The description of the population leaves the impression that a relatively deprived group of women were being used as subjects for this research project. This study's ethical credentials also merit attention. First, some of the women recruited were as young as 13 years. This raises questions about the ability of such young people to give consent to participation in research, especially at such a stressful time. Additionally, recruitment and randomisation happened after admission in labour when the woman's cervix had reached 3–4 cm dilatation. The possibility of truly informed consent under these circumstances is questionable (AIMS/NCT, 1997).

The researchers conclude that the care of the woman in labour should be reassessed in the light of these findings. Hodnett (2000c: 18) observes correctly that the conditions under which these women were expected to labour and give birth had more in common with the 'developing world' than with modern obstetric practice. Thus, she implies that the original aim of the study, to ascertain whether the central American findings are relevant in more sophisticated settings, has not been achieved by this study. This criticism may have been intended to endorse the research credentials of her Toronto study (Hodnett & Osborn, 1989a, b). On the basis of these data it is necessary to question whether the doula did anything more than compensate for a less than human environment for labour and birth. It may be suggested that the reassessment recommended by Kennell and colleagues (1991) should encompass not only the care of the woman in labour but also the wider environment of that care, including the built environment, the nursing care and the obstetric management.

Lay women without training

In her critique of the four earliest randomised controlled trials of support in labour, Hodnett (1997) emphasises their limited relevance to developed countries.

This criticism was intended to reflect more favourably on those studies undertaken in North America (see previous section). By scrutinising these studies, which also share the common feature that untrained lay women were the supporters, it is possible to assess the validity of Hodnett's criticism.

The RCT by Sosa and colleagues (1980) drew on an anthropological orientation to justify the assessment of the benefits of labour support on mother–infant interaction. The input of Klaus and Kennell into this study is clearly apparent, as it followed shortly after their well-known, but questionably authoritative, work on 'bonding' (Klaus & Kennell, 1976). Although the researchers reported that they planned to study the duration of labour, they later admitted that the effects of support on the length of labour were 'unexpected' (Klaus *et al.*, 1986; DONA, 1999).

This study was the first of two to be undertaken in the Social Security Hospital in Guatemala City in Guatemala. That the women who gave birth in this unit were relatively affluent is suggested by the fact that maternity care was financed through deduction of the costs from an employee's pay packet. This observation is supported by the researchers' description of the woman as healthier than the woman who attended the free public hospitals. The maternity unit was large. The researchers report an average of 60 births in 24 hours, indicating an annual number of births of almost 30 000. Because of the large numbers and due to lack of space since the earthquake four years earlier, no family member or continuous caretaker was permitted entry into the labour room. The routine practice for the care of the labouring woman involved infrequent vaginal examinations (VEs), auscultation of the fetal heart and help at birth. The researchers do not detail the frequency of the VEs or the nature of the help at the birth. In addition, the woman who was recruited into the experiment group received continuous support from an untrained lay woman. The support was provided from the time of admission to the birth. The support was in the form of physical contact, such as hand holding or back rubbing, conversation and a friendly, although previously unknown, presence.

First time mothers were recruited in labour, and recruitment continued until there were 20 in each arm of the trial. In the event of complications, such as prolonged labour, the woman was removed from the study. In order to complete recruitment of these 20 women, who achieved uncomplicated births, it was necessary for the researchers to recruit 103 women into the control group and 33 into the experimental group. Mother–baby interaction was observed during 45 minutes of skin to skin contact. The researchers are able to conclude that the woman in the control group was significantly more likely to experience a longer labour. This conclusion is drawn in spite of their data only referring to the time from the woman's admission to the birth. The experimental group were found to be significantly more likely to stroke, smile and talk to the newborn baby.

Sosa and colleagues suggest that the production of catecholamines due to stimulation of the autonomic nervous system by anxiety in labour may account for the less positive experiences among the control group. The unsupportive labour environment is held to be partly to blame, as it was crowded and unfamiliar and the women were unlikely to have been prepared through childbirth education classes. The researchers contemplate whether a family member, if permitted, would be able to produce similar beneficial results. They conclude by recommending the companionship of an untrained person as a low cost intervention which may reduce the length of labour as well as both maternal and neonatal problems. Thus, the advantages of this untrained person are explicitly recognised; this is because the costs of employing her were not inflated by the costs of training her, as would apply to, for example, a nurse. Similarly, it may be assumed that the benefits to the woman and her infant could also be associated with reduced costs due to the reduction in perinatal problems and the associated treatments. To whom the financial costs of perinatal problems accrue is not explained. It may be that they fall to the institution providing the maternity service. Thus the financial benefits of the doula to the health care system were apparent from the very first introduction of this concept.

A largely unchanged research team (Klaus *et al.*, 1986) undertook an extended replication study of that reported by Sosa and colleagues (1980). The research setting was also unchanged from that described above. Again, the recruitment and randomisation of first time mothers in labour featured. Women were eligible if cervical dilatation had reached 3 cm or less. Random allocation of the 465 eligible women led to an experimental group of 186 and a control group of 279, although once women with complications were excluded, the groups were reduced to 168 and 247 respectively. As in the earlier study, the intervention comprised the allocation of an untrained Guatemalan woman to give social support from the time of admission to the birth. The support comprised both emotional and physical elements and manifested itself as back rubbing, hand holding, explanation and encouragement. A difference from the previous study was that the 'patient' was told that she would never be left alone during labour.

Again the duration of labour was an important variable, but in the published report there is no indication of how it was assessed. The experimental group, however, are reported as having experienced significantly ($p < 0.001$) shorter labours. The incidence of caesarean and of augmentation of labour was also significantly lower in the experimental group. The researchers clearly consider that the findings of the earlier and smaller study are confirmed and go on to show similarities between their findings and the benefits of the Dublin protocol. The conclusion is drawn that social support may have the benefit of reducing the likelihood of admission to the neonatal unit. Unfortunately, there is no indication of who the researchers believe may benefit from this.

A comparable environment was the setting for another RCT on support in labour, undertaken in the Coronation Hospital in Johannesburg, South Africa (Hofmeyr *et al.*, 1991; Hofmeyr & Nikodem, 1996). This university/state hospital served a low income or 'mixed race' urban community which is described as being 'politically disadvantaged'. The question was posed as to whether company in labour, even though it was not ideal company, carries any benefits. The researchers anticipated that if suboptimal company proved beneficial, then more ideal company would be that much more effective.

In the research setting many of those who gave birth were young unmarried mothers. Additionally, the women seem to have been unsupported, as the authors state that the company of a support person was unusual. Unlike the other research settings, in Johannesburg there does not appear to have been any prohibition on companions. The intervention comprised support by an untrained lay woman, which was limited to the period after recruitment and randomisation in labour and up to the birth. The intention was that only social support in labour was to be provided. Each morning women were recruited if they were in established labour and the cervix was not more than 6 cm dilated. The experimental group comprised 92 first time mothers and the control group included 97 similar women. Data were collected by hourly specimens of blood being taken for catecholamine levels in labour and questionnaires being applied on day one and then six weeks and one year later.

The women who were recruited as the labour companions were chosen partly because they had no medical or nursing background, as this was deemed to be potentially alienating. Recruitment of the companions was via local churches. The involvement was essentially voluntary with only nominal expenses being paid at the rate of approximately £3 per day. Two labour supporters were selected by interview and role play, in an attempt to assess 'warmth of personality and ability to convey feelings of empathy' (Hofmeyr & Nikodem, 1996: 92). Two other women were also chosen to act as reserves, of whom one became involved. Like the Houston study by Kennell and colleagues (1991), all three of the labour supporters recruited were older women with children of their own. The labour companion was chosen to be of a 'similar background' (Hofmeyr & Nikodem, 1996: 92) to the woman, as she was considered less intimidating and easier to relate to than the nurse. The supporter was not previously known to the woman. Hofmeyr and Nikodem offered no formal training to the supporters, just an explanation of what was expected of them. The supporters were instructed to use their personal resources by being present, by talking and by holding – thus touch emerges once more. The supporter was also to focus on comfort, reassurance and praise in order to create a supportive environment which would sustain and possibly increase the labouring woman's self-confidence. These forms of support were to be provided as continuously as possible, but as the labour supporter was not permitted to stay after dark it is necessary to question the extent of the continuity of support.

The data showed a difference in the duration of labour, but it did not reach a significant level. The psychosocial effects were more markedly beneficial. These benefits included a positive labour experience and also lower state anxiety. The data collected at six weeks showed that in the supported group self-esteem was higher, parenting skills and personal relationships were better, there was less depression and breast feeding duration was longer. At 12 months the same general picture emerged, but the differences were no longer statistically significant. This study shows the possibility of long term effects attributable to a supportive birth environment. As Hodnett (1997) has also argued, these researchers suggest that nursing and midwifery staff may not be the ideal birth companions. This is because staff may be too busy, which is likely with more than one woman to attend, to be able to provide uninterrupted companionship. Hofmeyr and Nikodem also suggest that woman may be in awe of professional staff, which may be aggravated by the staff's relative youth.

On the basis of these findings Hofmeyr and Nikodem suggest that lay workers have a valuable role to contribute to the supportive care of the woman in labour. This conclusion should be interpreted in the context of their observation that 'nursing and midwifery staff may be too busy with nursing functions ... to provide companionship' (Hofmeyr & Nikodem, 1996: 97). This is a sad reflection on the midwife's priorities. Unlike many of the studies of support in labour these researchers provide minimal information on the environment of labour, referring only to 'a familiar community hospital' (Hofmeyr & Nikodem, 1996: 91). Although this account may sound convincing, the authors' anxieties about the risks of gastroenteritis due to formula feeding resonate more with a third world scenario. Thus, the reader is left, yet again, with an impression of an intervention which serves only to ameliorate the abysmal conditions of giving birth which are ordinarily available to the woman.

The 'politically disadvantaged' women of Johannesburg (Hofmeyr & Nikodem, 1996) may have certain features in common with the childbearing women of Botswana (Madi *et al.*, 1999), in that both groups were experiencing huge societal upheavals. In Botswana the traditional arrangement is for the birth attendant (TBA) and the mother's family to provide continuous support and encouragement throughout labour. Until the child is about three months old further intensive support is given by a responsible female relative. This arrangement is contrasted with the current pattern of hospital birth there, which excludes supportive relatives and, due to the pressure on staff, leaves the woman unaccompanied. Madi and colleagues, therefore, aimed to investigate the effects of the continuous presence of a known female companion providing support in labour in Botswana.

These researchers present a picture of labour and delivery care in a free maternity unit in which there are approximately 4000 births per year. The first time mother is usually, for cultural reasons, unmarried. The population was largely subsistence farmers. Labour and birth occurred in multi-occupancy rooms among staff, each of whom would be attending approximately four women in labour.

Recruitment and randomisation in labour resulted in an experiment group of 53 women and a control group of 56. Data were collected from the obstetric records after the birth. The researchers found that in the experiment group caesarean, vacuum extraction, analgesia use, amniotomy and oxytocin use were significantly lower than in the control group ($p < 0.05$). The researchers consider that the effects of the unsupportive hospital environment are likely to have been culturally moderated by the presence of the supportive female relative. Additionally, the relative's presence is thought likely to have prevented early interventions in the supported woman's labour and the 'cascade' which may ensue. Madi and colleagues suggest that the relative's presence may have produced other, indirect, effects. This may have involved the staff being 'freed up' to give more attention, by which is meant interventions, to the control group women as the experiment women were accompanied and not in need of such attention. The researchers also suggest that the presence of the relative may have applied implicit pressure on the woman in labour to 'behave' by not demanding attention and/or intervention.

While suggesting the benefits of an untrained yet intimately known support person, this study raises a number of issues. Madi and colleagues reflect a dismal picture of the care provided in labour, where staff are grossly overstretched and the only form of attention possible is obstetric intervention. Yet again, however, the reader is left with the abiding impression of a highly medicalised yet understaffed labour and delivery area. There is only one possible result of the introduction of the companion into this environment – merely to ameliorate the potentially iatrogenic management of uncomplicated labour and birth.

The non-institutional birth environment

The research on the supportive nature of the environment for labour and birth has addressed a range of institutional birth environments. This research has clearly demonstrated the interventions which are effective in reducing the hostile and unsupportive nature of these settings. I have not been able to refer to any research that focuses on birth environments other than the institutional because research on the benefits of that most supportive of birth environments, the woman's own home, has yet to be undertaken.

Conclusion

The impression which emerges from the research undertaken to investigate the effects of support in labour is clear: abysmal birthing environments being rendered less hostile by the endeavours of a kind-hearted woman companion. The environment has been shown to include a range of characteristics. Invariably the obstetric management is routinised and interventive. The nursing or midwifery service tends to be medically dominated. The nursing or midwifery service is likely to be understaffed, but if not staff are inattentive. The woman is prevented from or at least discouraged from enjoying the company of her own loved ones. The built environment features inappropriate spaces and a lack of privacy. In such dire conditions it should be no surprise that any intervention is effective in improving the woman's birth experience. A similar sentiment is articulated by

Robinson (1998: 20) when she observes in her commentary on Campero *et al.* (1998):

> '...a small dose of a prophylactic emotional antibiotic in a setting which is psychologically toxic.'

Robinson continues by suggesting that the support person or doula would not make much difference if the maternity unit offered a service which was in any way acceptable.

Robinson's critique of the research literature on support in labour is carried further by Odent (1996). He argues that the woman in labour is well-equipped to achieve a healthy and satisfactory birth experience, but only if she is not disturbed by the type of care which was formerly known as 'meddlesome' but is now termed interventive. He proposes that in providing care in labour the maxim should be 'leave well alone'. This maxim comprises the essence of the role of the midwife. Hers is fundamentally a 'watching brief'. Most of the research to which I have referred, though, has been undertaken in countries without a tradition of midwifery – obvious examples are Canada (Shields, 1978) or USA (Kennell *et al.*, 1991) – or with a tradition of midwifery which has been overtaken by medicalisation, such as Mexico (Campero *et al.*, 1998) or Botswwana (Madi *et al.*, 1999). Thus, it is necessary to question, as Hodnett and Osborn (1989a) did in relation to the Guatemalan studies, whether the studies reported here are generalisable to the UK situation.

It may be that Odent's argument could be further advanced by considering why such support is so effective. The answer may be found in the iatrogenic effects of the medicalisation of birth. The removal of the control of labour away from the woman and her body into the hands of our medical colleagues has left the woman without her usual resources on which to fall back. Examples would be her family, her usual birth attendants and her feeling that she, in the form of her body, is confident of the ability to give birth. Thus, the traditional form of care has been eliminated. It has been supplanted by a form of management to which the term 'aggressive' is not uncommonly applied (O'Regan, 1998). It is suggested that this form of management may only be rendered less than iatrogenic by the introduction of an entirely new member of staff – to whom we give our attention in the next chapter.

Chapter 6
The doula

Having examined, in Chapter 5, the research evidence which alerts us to the need for a supportive environment in labour, it is now appropriate to study the person who has been recommended to ensure this environment (Hodnett, 2000c: 7). Because it is a term which I introduced to this book in Chapter 5 and because it is widely used, especially in the North American literature, I refer to this person as the 'doula'. Thus, this chapter begins with a reflection on the meaning of this term. I then move on to contemplate the services which the doula provides and her background. This section makes further use of the research studies already outlined in Chapter 5. After going on to consider what the doula does not do, an analysis of the significance of the appearance of the doula on the maternity care scene follows. This is combined with an assessment of the rationale for her existence. Finally, I give some attention to the implications of the introduction of the doula for systems of maternity care, for those involved in maternity care and, particularly, for the midwife.

Origins and meanings

In order to help us understand the reasons for her introduction, it may be useful to reflect on the origins and meaning of the term 'doula'. In an early RCT this term was introduced as having been used by Dana Raphael (1973) to signify a 'supportive companion' (Sosa *et al.*, 1980: 597). Raphael's anthropological study identified the widespread practice of 'a female of the same species' staying with the parturient through her labour and the birth. In human beings Raphael states that this companion is a family member or friend. She suggests that this companion's continued presence with the mother and baby makes a crucial contribution to the long term success of breast feeding. The term is introduced in this way (Raphael, 1973: 24):

> 'We have adopted a word to describe the person who performs this [supportive] function – the *doula*.'

The term is explained by Raphael with a cursory reference to 'Aristotle's time'. Further limited enlightenment is found in the acknowledgement of 'Eleni Rassias for the word "doula"' (Raphael, 1973: 10), although there is no other indication of its origin. The meaning that Raphael attaches to this term is made abundantly clear in a later publication dwelling on the long term nature of the doula's help which, by definition, follows the labour and birth (Raphael, 1988).

On the basis of Raphael's observations and a fleeting reference to the doula, the first Guatemalan RCT on support (Sosa *et al.*, 1980, see the section 'Lay women without training' in Chapter 5) proceeded to refer to her as a 'companion'. By 1986, though, the meaning of this term had been subtly amended. An almost unchanged research team undertook the second Guatemalan RCT (Klaus *et al.*, 1986). By this time, however, the word doula was being described as a Greek word meaning a 'woman's servant' (Klaus, 1986: 585). Reference is made to it having been used previously by Raphael (1973) to mean a woman helping the mother in the home after the birth.

Further refinement of the meaning of the term had happened by the time of the Houston study of support in labour (Kennell *et al.*, 1991). In this study there is no longer any reference to Raphael's anthropological study. The doula, however, had developed her role to become 'an experienced woman who guides and assists a new mother in her infant-care tasks' (Kennell *et al.*, 1991: 2198).

In view of the multiplicity of interpretations of this word I sought the advice of a Greek colleague who is a nurse. I was reliably informed 'the term doula is not used in childbearing in Greece. It refers to a maid with a very negative meaning' (Tzepapadaki, 2000, pers. comm.). Further investigation suggests that the origins of this word appear to relate to the slaves who were widely used among the more affluent members of Greek society during the fourth century BC. This interpretation is endorsed by an authoritative English–Greek dictionary: 'slave – δουλα' (Stavropoulos & Hornby, 1977: 637). This meaning is expanded by a more popular dictionary to differentiate the male slave 'δουλος' (doulos) from his female equivalent (Sideris, 1996: 313). Thus, the 'negative meaning' to which my colleague referred becomes abundantly clear. The least offensive meaning for 'δουλα' is found in Sideris' (1996: 490) interpretation of the word as meaning 'maid, servant'.

For the person referred to in the support literature, 'παραμανα' (paramana) would be the preferred term (Sideris, 1996: 687). The 'paramana' is a lay woman who remains with the woman and is alongside her during her labour and stays with her afterwards to help her. The help provided even extends as far as acting as a wet-nurse. Thus, Sideris' translation of this word to mean 'nanny' becomes most apposite.

The usual current use of the term doula is found in an old Greek proverb which distinguishes the capabilities necessary in the person with whom a man shares his life and his home. This proverb implies that this ideal person should be both practical and presentable. Thus the practical, but low status, doula is contrasted with the more ideal woman, who should also be presentable. This implies that the doula is in no way ladylike (Tzepapadaki, 2000, pers. comm.): 'The good housewife is both doula and lady'.

From this scrutiny it becomes apparent that the word doula probably originated with ancient Greek society. Further, even in the most non-politically correct sections of Greek society, the word is no longer used to describe a person as the meaning conveyed is too derogatory. This etymological background serves to shed a new light on the rationale for the doula and on the relationship between the doula and the woman in labour. The doula clearly originated from a menial person whose role, far from being supportive, sisterly and with the woman, comprised little more than unthinking – even slavish – obedience.

This contrast bears comparison with the care provider who may share certain attributes in common with the person introduced as the modern 'doula'. This is the midwife. At one extreme, there is the Dutch midwife who is often regarded as the epitome of high occupational status (Mander, 1995). By way of contrast, the reverse may apply in India where the *dâi* performs some of the functions of a midwife. Her status, however, may be too lowly even to deserve the title 'midwife'. This is because her role relates in the main part to minimising the dangerous pollution which is perceived to be associated with childbirth (Jeffery *et al.*, 1989).

In view of this scrutiny of the etymological background of the 'doula', the question which emerges is 'why?'. The rationale for the introduction of a less than accurate Greek term, when an appropriate Old English word 'midwife' exists, is unclear. It is necessary to consider the North American culture into which the doula was introduced. As mentioned in Chapter 2 the virtual extinction of the midwife there by the medical establishment is relatively recent (Jackson & Mander, 1995). Perhaps for reasons like this, the term may still be less than acceptable.

The doula's characteristics

Having reached some understanding of how and why this term is used, it is now appropriate to consider what the doula does and the nature of her personal background which enables her to do it. In order to consider these aspects, I draw mainly on the research literature. Additionally, I supplement this by reference to the material which has been produced in order to provide information for the potential client.

The activities of the doula

The primary aim of the doula is to provide social support for the woman in labour. While support is generally considered to be empowering, in this context there is an additional dimension. The term which is frequently used to explain the doula role is 'mothering the mother' (Raphael, 1981; Klaus *et al.*, 1993; Stansfield, 1997). This term, by suggesting that the woman in labour is less than fully adult, carries overtones of condescension and 'maternalism'. I suggest that this attitude may not be entirely appropriate towards a woman undergoing the transition to parenthood.

Support in labour, such as that offered by the doula, tends to be defined in terms of four general aspects (McNiven *et al.*, 1992):

(1) Physical comfort
(2) Emotional support
(3) Instruction and/or information
(4) Advocacy.

As these general aspects of support have been examined in Chapter 1, I make no further explicit reference to them here. I begin by examining the specific activities or behaviours which have been allocated to or assumed by the doula.

Presence

The issue of the presence of the support person may at first sight appear too obvious to be worth mentioning. This is reflected in occasional derogatory phrases, such as 'mere physical presence' (O'Driscoll *et al.*, 1993: 93) or 'just being there' (Sleutel, 2000: 39). This concept, however, is fundamentally important to care, particularly in labour (Siddiqui, 1999). Following her research on competencies among expert nurses, Benner (1984) was able to define presence in terms of being with, as opposed to doing for, the person. This definition resonates powerfully with the original Old English meaning of the word 'midwife', which essentially refers to someone who is 'with woman' (Macdonald, 1981).

The concept of presence as supportive emerged clearly in an RCT on intervention in labour (Lavender *et al.*, 1999). As part of the study, these researchers collected data relating to positive and negative aspects of labour, by using a questionnaire with open items. The women in each of the three trial arms found good support to be a most important and beneficial aspect of their labour. This support was provided by both the midwife and partner or friend. The supportive nature of the presence of even a relatively inactive companion manifests itself in quotations, such as:

'I don't think I could have coped if I'd been alone.'

(Lavender *et al.*, 1999: 42)

In a study of support in labour by Shields (1978), the presence of the nurse was found to be the aspect of supportive care most frequently mentioned by the new mother (*n* = 20, 25%). As mentioned in Chapter 5, though, the methodology was of a questionable quality The benefits of another's presence emerged marginally more convincingly in the study by Sosa and colleagues (1980). In this first major RCT on support in labour, the company of an albeit untrained and unknown companion in labour, was serendipitously found to be associated with shorter labour. These findings were endorsed by a full-scale replication study in a more technologically advanced environment in Houston, Texas (Kennell *et al.*, 1991). The importance of presence was affirmed by the fact that this observer may not even have been visible to the woman in labour. Thus, Kennell *et al.* (1991: 2201) are able to conclude:

'it is impressive that part of [the companion's] effect may be solely her presence.'

An RCT in Mexico City was organised along broadly similar lines, but without producing the same marked reduction in the levels of medical intervention (Campero *et al.*, 1998). The significant psychosocial benefits for the supported women, however, are attributed by the researchers to the doula's continuous presence. A Finnish study (Tarkka & Paunonen, 1996) served to raise an issue which is likely to emerge as increasingly important. This is the relative benefit of the presence of the support person, compared with that of the woman's partner or friend. These researchers found that the woman's experience of labour caused the partner's presence to matter less than the professional's. By way of contrast, in the study by Madi *et al.* (1999) support was by a female relative, rather than a professional. This intervention resulted in certain indirect benefits of a supportive presence; for example, the supported women not 'demanding' attention which inevitably and invariably took the form of intervention. Additionally, because of the staff not needing to show their attention to the supported women by applying interventions, the control group may have experienced the dubious benefits of even more interventions.

A USA trained doula describes her role in terms of the importance of the initial assessment of the woman's needs (Stansfield, 1997). On the basis of this, she describes how 'simply being there' (Stansfield, 1997: 8) may be all that is necessary. She expands this point in a way that resonates with the findings of Kennell and colleagues (1991): at times just sitting in the room quietly, remaining calm and peaceful is all that some women want (Stansfield, 1997: 8). A variation on this theme is the emphasis in the doula literature on her being available in the early stages of labour by telephone contact (Klaus *et al.*, 1993: 18). Thus, the question of the value of her availability as a substitute for her actual physical presence emerges.

Continuity

The continuity of the support person's presence has also been suggested as interesting, or even important. In Hodnett's systematic review (2000c) this aspect is regarded as crucial, although the rationale is not altogether clear. The assumption has been made that continuity of presence is a precise proxy for effective support. This assumption has resulted in studies of nurses' activities, utilising work sampling techniques, being used to assess the level of support offered to women in labour (McNiven *et al.*, 1992; Gagnon & Waghorn, 1996). The accuracy of this assumption is uncertain to say the least.

In an intervention study by Gagnon and colleagues (1997) the duration and continuity of the presence of the nurse was strictly enforced. This resulted in a high level of continuity of the nurse's presence, which was unheard of in the Canadian labour and delivery setting. Continuity of the doula's presence was also found helpful in the Mexico City study (Campero *et al.*, 1998). In other studies, such as Kennell and colleagues (1991), the doula was required to remain at the woman's bedside from admission until the birth. Whether this is strictly and literally accurate is not possible to assess from the data provided. The account by Hofmeyr and Nikodem (1996), however, may be more enlightening. These researchers, probably in view of the civil unrest in South Africa at the time, did not require the doula to remain after nightfall; thus continuity was somewhat limited.

A realistic recommendation for the continuity of the support person's presence emerges most appropriately from the study by Shields (1978). This researcher was able to conclude that the level of continuity is best determined by the needs or otherwise of the woman in labour. Thus, it may be that a more important aspect than rigid continuity is not just the physical presence, but the perceived support or availability of the person in attendance.

The literature for the prospective client emphasises very strongly the likelihood of the doula offering continuity of support (Simkin & Way, 1998). This is summarised:

> 'Perhaps the most crucial role of the doula is providing continuous emotional reassurance and comfort.'
>
> (DONA, 1999: 1)

This ability may reflect the doula's unique selling point, in contrast to the staff who provide more wide-ranging care (Simkin & Way, 1998). Klaus and colleagues (1993) endorse the doula's role by drawing attention to the pressures on staff in the labour and delivery area. They go on to observe the all too obvious limitations of the father in meeting the needs of the woman in labour. These authors then raise the possibility that some maternity units are able to provide one-to-one care and in such conditions a member of staff is able to act as the doula. This statement, however, carries a warning which will prove disconcerting:

> 'in most cases . . . midwives generally care for several patients at any one time'.
>
> (Klaus *et al.*, 1993: 11)

One-to-one care

The concept of continuity suggests that each labouring woman is supported by one person. It is necessary to consider the corollary of this arrangement, that is, that each member of staff cares for only one woman. That this may not be the case emerged very clearly in the RCT by Madi and colleagues (1999). These researchers reported a staff to woman ratio of one to four. Thus any possibility of one-to-one care was excluded. It may be assumed that this ratio refers to midwifery staff; if it refers to total staff, the situation is even more dire. The Dublin regime claims to ensure one-to-one care by the allocation of an individual member of staff or student to an individual 'patient' (O'Driscoll *et al.*, 1993: 93). The doula's 'mission statement' by Klaus and colleagues (1993: 97) praises the benefits of the Dublin regime. While ignoring the more interventive aspects of the

Dublin package which O'Driscoll and colleagues (1993: 94) believe make it possible, Klaus *et al.* propose that the supportive relationship for the woman in labour is worth imitating. Clearly the doula's advocates emphasise the likelihood of the midwife or nurse caring for a number of women (Klaus *et al.*, 1993: 18) to serve their own purposes. These ends would not be advanced by explaining that the reason for the midwife working in this way is not through choice, but because of the medicalised system of maternity care within which she is all too often employed.

Empathy

The aspects of the supportive relationship which have been mentioned already should serve to create the ideal emotional environment in which empathetic support is likely to be offered. The Johannesburg study was the RCT which explicitly sought empathy in the women supporters who were recruited. The interviewers were seeking in the volunteers 'warmth of personality and ability to convey feelings of empathy' (Hofmeyr & Nikodem, 1996: 92).

The ability to easily develop an empathetic relationship is part of the job description for the doula (Klaus *et al.*, 1993: 18). But these authors regard this ability as innate and natural, rather than one which requires a high standard of learned communication skills. They further suggest that an empathetic approach in the doula is more likely if she has personal experience of childbearing. Klaus and colleagues further draw on the Dublin regime to show the easy benefits of empathy. Describing the support person in Dublin as a 'midwife' Klaus *et al.* (1993: 98) recount how she 'practises her craft with skill, caring and intuitive and experienced knowledge'.

Clinical functions

The research studies detailed in Chapter 5, with the exception of occasional blurring, generally differentiate the support personnel who undertake clinical tasks from those who do not. The literature on the doula invariably falls into the latter category (Simkin & Way, 1998: 1; DONA, 1999: 1). The example which features considerable 'blurring' is the Dublin protocol (O'Driscoll *et al.*, 1993). The authors maintain that the support person is required to distinguish the emotional support which she or he provides, from the clinical activities which they also undertake. This double function might be perceived as challenging, especially if the support person is not qualified, as the Dublin support person may not be (O'Driscoll *et al.*, 1993: 102). The authors are reassuring that these demands may easily be met. This assertion would be more credible if the clinical functions, such as observation of the vital signs, are actually made only as infrequently as the stated 'intervals of two hours' (O'Driscoll *et al.*, 1993: 93). It is clear that such infrequent observations would certainly allow the support person time to concentrate on supporting. Such infrequent recordings, however, may cause concern to those who are aware of the iatrogenic effects of the interventions which the Dublin regime advocates to augment labour.

The distinction between the clinical functions of the support person and their social functions may be more apparent than real (Keirse *et al.*, 1989). While the individual supporter may be clear about the demands on their support at any given time, the perceptions or expectations of their colleagues may differ. The likelihood of tensions arising in situations featuring such conflicting demands emerges in the American case study by Sleutel (2000). The subject of the case study clearly and appropriately regards her primary loyalty as being to the woman whom she is attending. The medical personnel, who in that setting are said to be ultimately responsible for the woman's care, may be operating to a different agenda. In this way support may become secondary to other, possibly technological or medical, imperatives.

The contrast with this dual and potentially conflicting responsibility may be used as another 'unique selling point' by those who advocate the introduction of the doula. The focus of the doula on the non-clinical aspects of the care of the labouring woman is invariably emphasised:

> 'Doulas specialise in non-medical skills and do not perform clinical tasks, such as vaginal exams or fetal heart rate monitoring.'
>
> (Simkin & Way, 1998: 1)

This may be contrasted with other care providers such as the midwife, whose role is described merely in terms of ensuring 'the safe passage of the mother and baby' (Simkin & Way, 1998: 1). Simkin appears to emphasise what she regards as a shortcoming in the midwife and, in so doing, may aggravate the anxieties of the woman contemplating labour:

> 'When compared to nurses and midwives who have clinical responsibilities that have to take priority over the mother's emotional needs, the doula can always remain beside the woman...'
>
> (Simkin in Hanson, 2000a: 2)

This account leaves those of us who are midwives with a certain feeling of *déjà vu*. This arises because being with the mother is a crucial and not inconsiderable part of the role of the midwife (Kirkham, 1989). Whether Simkin's interpretation of the relationship is accurate and, if so, how it has come to be will be addressed in the section 'The significance of the doula' later in this chapter.

In spite of the emphasis on the non-clinical role of the doula, this role may be adopted less than strictly. That the doula may occasionally step outside her non-clinical remit is apparent in the words of Simkin in a published interview (Hanson, 2000a):

> 'But [the woman in labour] also needs someone with a perspective on when to throw in the towel, and to recognise that this is not going normally, or that we need some interventions here.'

There is no doubt that the someone to whom Simkin is referring is the doula.

Non-verbal signals

Non-verbal messages are crucial to ensuring effective communication, but they may also have the reverse effect. According to Schott and Henley (1996: 72), due to such signals being based on cultural conventions, misinterpretation may give rise to serious offence. In their examples of non-verbal communication these authors include 'eye contact, facial expressions, head/body movements/posture, gestures, touch and physical distance' (Schott & Henley, 1996: 72).

Physical distance/proximity and touch

The appropriate use of closeness and physical contact are widely regarded in the literature as an indicator of emotional contact, support and empathy. The cultural background of the people involved as well as the nature of their relationship influences the proximity with which they feel comfortable. The social rules about acceptable touch are gender-based, situation specific and culture bound. These rules also regulate which body part may be touched, when and by whom. In labour physical contact may take the form of hand holding, or hugs, or activities with some obvious intended benefit, such as back rubbing. The reduction of distance between the woman and her support person may be achieved by sitting, standing or walking alongside her.

The cultural dimensions of proximity and touch emerged clearly in the study by Holroyd and colleagues (1997) (see Chapter 5). This study was undertaken in Hong Kong among ethnic Chinese women, whose culture disdains close proximity and touch by strangers. Obviously some other cultural groups may interpret personal space in very different terms. It may fit our cultural stereotypes that Hispanic women in Texas and Mexican women were happy with physical proximity and contact (Kennell *et al.*, 1991; Campero *et al.*, 1998). The observation, however, that an overwhelmingly white sample of midwestern women found touch acceptable to the point of being therapeutic may be surprising (Birch, 1986: 272).

Touch is one of a repertoire of techniques reported by Stansfield (1998) as being used in her practice as a doula and she combines it with other physical interventions, such as massage. In a review claiming the 'rediscovery of an essential ingredient of childbirth' Klaus and Kennell (1997: 1034) explain the beneficial effects of the doula's touch. Citing, but not referencing Uvnäs-Moberg, general touch is claimed to stimulate oxytocin production. Klaus and Kennell further maintain that this hormone gives rise to drowsiness, euphoria and an increased ability to tolerate pain.

Eye contact

In the same way as their ethnic Chinese sample sought to avoid physical proximity, Holroyd and colleagues (1997) found that eye contact was unwelcome. This is because it is regarded as disrespectful and rude (Schott & Henley, 1996: 72). Other cultures may regard too little eye contact as discourteous and evasive, whereas northern Europeans seek to tread a fine line between the two. The maintenance of eye contact was one of the techniques taught to the doulas by Campero and colleagues (1998) and appreciated by Swedish women (Lundgren & Dahlberg, 1998). Continuing direct eye contact is one of the mainstays of the Dublin regime. Its importance, however, appears to be more related to preventing the dreaded eye-closing than establishing empathy (O'Driscoll *et al.*, 1993).

The experience of Stansfield (1997) lends further support to the use of eye contact. She uses what she describes as 'close eye contact, when the going gets tough' (p. 66) in order to enhance the woman's ability to retain her self control.

Reassurance

Although widely dismissed as paternalistic in comparison with information giving, reassurance is commended as one of the activities by which the doula supports the woman in labour. It emerged as one of the helpful aspects of emotional support in the one-to-one study by Gagnon and colleagues (1997). Reassurance was also encouraged as one of the interventions to be used by the doula to raise the labouring woman's flagging self-confidence (Hofmeyr & Nikodem, 1996).

'Emotional reassurance' may, according to Doulas of North America (DONA, 1999), be the most crucial role of the doula, while Stansfield (1997) uses it to help keep the mother relaxed and to encourage the father's participation. Reassurance is adjusted to become 'firm' when Klaus and colleagues (1993) implement their modification of the Dublin regime of support.

Supporting the father

It is usual to assume that support in labour is offered only to the woman who is in labour. It may be helpful, though, to consider this issue in broader terms as there is an increasing awareness of the psychosocial needs of the father in relation to childbearing. Draper (1997) recognises that the male partner is present during labour, not only to support the woman but also to meet his own needs as he becomes a father. Thus, he too is likely to require the support of health care providers.

The role envisaged for the father in relation to the doula emerges clearly in the book by Klaus and colleagues (1993). This material presents a picture of North American childbearing which may be the corollary of the work sampling studies described in Chapter 5. Klaus and colleagues (1993: 5) emphasise the crucial role of the father in providing all the basic care necessary for the woman in labour. The assumption is clearly that the father is the ideal person to help the woman find a comfortable position, to provide her with fluids to drink and to attend to her personal hygiene. Whether this assumption applies in other settings outside North America is a matter for conjecture. On the basis of this assumption, however, Klaus and colleagues argue that this form of caretaking, which is all that is available to the woman during the nurse's lengthy absences, is not adequate. These authors argue that the woman also needs a nurturing experienced person who is able to provide a reassuring and constant presence in addition to the father's care. These two kinds of support, it is argued, serve to complement each other. The father's far from insignificant role in providing basic care in the labour/delivery area is repeatedly emphasised; an example is the way that the usual care involves only the father being present with the woman between the visits by the nurse or the physician (Klaus et al., 1993: 9). It may not be surprising that this level of responsibility may at least be 'challenging' to some fathers. Klaus and colleagues (1993: 21) go on to discuss the unsurprising tendency for the father to back away from over involvement in the woman's care. When this happens these authors recognise an opportunity for the doula to move in closer to her.

This impression of much of the care of the labouring woman being provided by the father is endorsed by Klaus and Kennell (1997: 1035), who claim that 'fathers provide support to about 80% of labouring women' in the USA. Because of the father's sterling work these authors consider that the doula may be regarded as unnecessary. At this juncture, however, the father's shortcomings are recognised in terms of his 'not being well prepared' (Klaus & Kennell, 1997: 1035). This recognition serves to highlight the need for the services of the doula. Due only to her presence the father is not left as the 'responsible person' caring for the labouring woman. The strengths of this 'perfect support team for the woman' are widely endorsed (DONA, 1999: 2; Gilliland, 1998). The impression of a large majority of care in labour being provided by the expectant father may be disconcerting to those accustomed to different systems of health care. The recommendation that his care should be superseded by that of a relatively untrained person is only marginally less so.

The doula's background

On the basis of the research outlined in Chapter 5, it is becoming apparent that the need for the specific interventions offered by the doula is the product of a system of maternity care in which certain assumptions are fundamental. These assumptions, such as the reliance on the father to provide care and the overwhelming medicalisation of labour and birth (Sleutel, 2000), may be disconcertingly alien to other health care systems. In order to provide a more complete picture of the person who offers these services, it may be helpful to examine the personal and occupational characteristics which make up her background.

Duration of relationship with the woman

The importance of there being an established relationship between the woman and the person who supports her in labour is uncertain (Hodnett, 2000b). Surprisingly, in the study by Rennie and colleagues (1998) even the known midwife was found to matter less during the birth than the woman anticipated. This lessening of the midwife's importance was in contrast to that of the partner, which increased significantly. The Canadian RCT (Hodnett & Osborn, 1989a, b) raises issues relating to how the pre-existing relationship is assessed. While claiming that the monitrice was 'familiar' or 'known' to the woman, this familiarity or knowledge was based on only having met each other twice during the pregnancy. It may be that this is more than the usual pattern of care, but to claim that the two 'know' each other may be something of an overstatement.

Two of the other RCTs (Kennell *et al.*, 1991; Sosa *et al.*, 1980) report the absence of any relationship, by stating that the doula was not previously known to the woman. On the basis of these RCTs Hodnett (1997: 80) is able to state:

> '... support by a woman who has no previous social bond ... has no known risks and has the potential to effect important improvements.'

On the other hand, the RCT by Madi and colleagues (1999) ensured that a relationship existed by enlisting the support of one of the woman's female relatives. This intervention was presented as an attempt to provide support which mirrored the traditional arrangement as closely as possible. In spite of the significant improvements identified in Madi and colleagues' study, the emphasis on the benefits of an unknown person continue to be advanced:

> 'Obstetric outcomes were most improved and intervention rates most dramatically lowered by doulas in settings where the women had no loved ones present.'
>
> (Simkin & Way, 1998: 3)

This impression of some uncertainty about the benefits of an established relationship is further confused by the quotation in the book by Klaus and colleagues (1993), which implies that the events at the birth are all that matter:

> 'The family is born in the delivery room – J Lind MD Stockholm.'

Just in case, though, the doula's role is defined as meeting the couple not more than three months prior to the expected date of the birth. In the same way as Hodnett and Osborn (1989a, b) had previously made assumptions about the benefits of these two or three contacts during pregnancy, they are regarded as sufficient to allow a relationship to be developed (Klaus *et al.*, 1993: 18).

Childbearing experience

The need for the attendant in childbirth to have given birth to a child or children is an ongoing topic of debate (Mander, 1996; Bewley, 1997). This characteristic may be assumed to indicate comparability of at least one aspect of the two people's background. Common values may also be assumed, thus facilitating a more supportive relationship. In the Houston RCT (Kennell *et al.*, 1991) the 11 women selected as doulas had given birth to at least one healthy child following an uncomplicated labour and vaginal birth. The authors omit to mention, however, whether this selection was deliberate or serendipitous or, if the former, the rationale for this criterion. Similarly, Hofmeyr and Nikodem (1996) recruited women who were mothers of grown up families to be supporters for the labouring women. Again, though, there is no indication of whether this selection was planned or fortuitous.

The more recent literature advising the woman about the doula gives the impression of being flexible in this respect. The DONA website describes doulas as 'being trained and experienced in childbirth, although they may or may not have given birth themselves' (DONA, 1999: 1). The earlier book by Klaus and colleagues (1993: 6) defines the doula as either 'an older experienced woman or a younger birthing woman'. Later in the same book the authors' real beliefs emerge when they write: 'Most doulas have delivered children of their own' (Klaus *et al.*, 1993. 18). The benefits are explained in terms of the resulting innate sense and natural empathy, although this is soon modified by the disclaimer that personal birthing experience is not essential. The situation becomes marginally clearer in the chapter on 'How to find and choose a doula'. After mentioning desirable personality factors, the authors write (1993: 127): 'Experience of childbirth, either personally and also through attendance at many births...' Thus, although, personal childbearing experience appears to matter in the doula, its precise influence is unclear.

Comparability of backgrounds

While the experience of having borne a child is of questionable significance, other similarities in the backgrounds of the supporter and the woman tend, at least in historical terms, to have been taken for granted (Loudon, 1992: 179). These similarities may adopt a number of different forms, such as gender and culture, some of which are discussed below. The study which most explicitly addressed this issue was the Johannesburg RCT (Hofmeyr & Nikodem, 1996). In this study the researchers chose the labour companions from the same back-ground as the labouring women. This was partly for the benefit of the research, to eliminate the possibility of any difference being due to 'nursing' interventions. The other reason for this choice related to what might be termed the 'accessibility' of the supporter. Hofmeyr & Nikodem (1996: 92) explain this in terms of the supporter being 'less intimidating and easier to relate to'. These authors go on to state that the 'medical approach' to childbearing tends to take over from the woman, perhaps intending reassurance but more likely achieving condescension. This may result in the woman in labour, especially if she is not affluent, feeling over-awed by the staff. Thus, the woman may be prevented from being able to accept a supportive relationship were it to be available.

These observations are endorsed by Hodnett (1997) in her critique of 'nurses' as labour supporters. She traces the working pattern of the nurse, based on the Canadian work-sampling studies. The social organisation of the nurse's working environment, Hodnett maintains, causes the nurse to adopt certain values which might be summarised as 'medical'. These include the nurse's confidence in 'obstetric technology' (Hodnett, 1997: 79). Additionally, the nurse comes, as a result of her socialisation, to value the more objective aspects of maternity care, such as the print-out from a cardiotocograph. This valuing of objectivity is contrasted with the woman's belief system. The woman is more likely to value the more 'subjective' aspects of childbearing; Hodnett's examples include the use of touch to convey either reassurance or the need for information. For these reasons, Hodnett argues that the nurse is not the appropriate person to provide support in labour.

Data have not been identified, and may not yet exist, to indicate whether this comparability of background applies to the doula currently in practice. No mention of the doula's background has been found in the material produced by her North American advocates.

Training/education

The preparation of the doula was addressed in detail in some of the RCTs. For example, in the study by Kennell and colleagues (1991) each of the doulas underwent what appears to have been a highly intensive three week course. At the end of this period the doula had been taught a wide range of material including abnormal labour, obstetric procedures and hospital policies. This curriculum must have been daunting and it is necessary to question the extent to which it had the effect of socialising the doula into the institution in which she practised. Alternatively, it may be necessary to surmise that the doula's orientation to childbearing would have been changed by exposure to this material. The first and second Guatemalan RCTs (Sosa *et al.*, 1980; Klaus *et al.*, 1986) involved women who were 'untrained', although no detail is provided about their characteristics or the criteria for their selection. In the Johannesburg RCT, on the other hand, Hofmeyr and Nikodem (1996) clearly spell out the advantages which they perceive are associated with the supporter's absence of training. In this RCT the supporters were given only 'a careful explanation of what was expected of them' (Hofmeyr & Nikodem, 1996: 92). These researchers regard education as having the potential to distance the supporter and to render her less effective (see the previous section) due to her relative 'inaccessibility'.

In the book by Klaus and colleagues (1993) an appendix is devoted to the 'training' of the doula. This section details the doula's background, which is likely to be as a childbirth educator, with home birth or lay midwifery, or as a woman who was thus supported in labour. The rationale for wishing to train as a doula is either that the woman may want to give something back or may wish to compensate for the deficiencies in the care she experienced. The 'basic training' (Klaus *et al.*, 1993: 137) is briefly described in terms of 'courses and actual experience'. The recommended reading features material by Simkin, by Perez, by Kitzinger and by Odent. The nature of the training is summarised as 'we believe that most of the training should center around hands-on experience' (Klaus *et al.*, 1993: 137).

This account of doula preparation leaves the reader with the definite impression that only training or an apprenticeship, rather than an education, is all that is necessary. The lack of any objectives or learning outcomes is disconcerting to an educationist. The possibility begins to emerge that this scenario may not just be uneducational, but that it may also be anti-educational. This anxiety is endorsed by the account of Doulas of North America of the training/certification programme (Simkin & Way, 1998: 5). The entry qualifications require only prior knowledge of childbirth. On entry into the programme there is an 'intensive two or three day seminar' (DONA, 1999). Certification as a doula follows background work, learning activities, observation of classes, reading and an assessment by a written examination or essay. Recommendations from clients, medical personnel, midwives and nurses are also required, although whether these are testimonials or confidential references is not clear.

The likelihood of a limited educational background is endorsed by Klaus and colleagues' (1993: 136) account. The training of the doula is required to meet minimum standards, but this is intended to facilitate communication only at a 'visceral' level. By way of comparison, 'Medical caregivers often communicate only at an intellectual level' (Klaus *et al.*, 1993: 136). This discussion of the appropriately named 'basic training' serves to reinforce the impression of an anti-intellectual, even anti-educational orientation.

Gender

My discussion of the doula only as a female is an accurate reflection of the literature. In her original work, Raphael (1973: 36) gave only cursory attention to the 'rare male doula'. She did, however, show that the grandfather of the baby has the potential to fulfil this role successfully (Raphael, 1973: 151). The emphasis on the female doula to the exclusion of any males persists (Klaus *et al.*, 1993). While the Dublin regime praises the ability of female nurses and midwives to empathise with the woman in labour, this does not preclude the male medical student from providing this form of support (O'Driscoll & Meagher, 1986: 88).

Loyalty

The loyalty of the doula is one of her characteristics which allows little scope for uncertainty. This loyalty to the woman is extended in some of the literature to the point of disparaging other care providers, such as Stansfield's (1997: 66) reference to nursing staff being 'so used' to intravenous infusions that they do not deserve a mention, or Simkin and Way (1998: 2) accusing others of ignoring the woman's psychosocial needs. Whereas Sleutel (2000) discussed her nurse-informant's uncertainty about where her loyalty should reside, the authors who focus on the doula face no such dilemma (Sagady, 1997). For this reason the doula may be regarded as infinitely preferable to her colleagues in more established occupational groups (Hofmeyr & Nikodem, 1996). As an employee of an institution, such as a maternity unit, Hodnett (1997) considers how the nurse's loyalty may be divided in a number of directions. While she recognises her potential by admitting that 'nurses can provide effective labour support' (Hodnett, 1997: 79), she goes on to detail the organisational and social factors in the labour and delivery area which serve to impede the effective provision of that support.

What the doula does not do

By examining the accounts in the RCTs and the other literature it has been possible to piece together a clear picture of who the doula is and what she does. It is now necessary to look closely at the other side of that coin. This involves contemplating those activities which the doula declines to undertake or is prevented from performing.

Much of the literature which is intended for those considering engaging a doula focuses on the activities from which the doula is debarred. At first sight this appears a wise precaution in view of what might be widespread uncertainty about this person and her functions. Some of this advice concentrates on the relationship between the doula and the woman and the ways in which effective support may be ensured. Examples of such advice are found in Raphael's original work, which recommends that the doula should never assume that she knows best and, for this reason, she should not give advice unless specifically asked to (Raphael, 1973: 160). This slightly retiring approach appears to differ from the recommendations of some practitioners, such as Stansfield (1997: 66) who states that as a doula she offers 'firm but gentle words of encouragement'. These comments are reminiscent of the Dublin regime's recommendation of 'a sense of firm reassurance, which is so sorely needed at this time' (O'Driscoll & Meagher, 1986: 93).

Further warnings are offered in Klaus and colleagues' book, which suggests that the doula should never panic and that she should not think about her own needs (Klaus *et al.*, 1993: 139). In stark contrast to the principles of active management of labour, these authors further recommend that the doula should take no account of how long the labour has been or is likely to be (Klaus *et al.*, 1993: 138). This counsel of perfection may be difficult to achieve in view of the emphasis of active management on 'progress' in labour as invariably dictated by the partograph (O'Driscoll & Meagher, 1993:44). As well as her supportive role, the doula's advocacy role begins to emerge when Klaus and colleagues recommend that not only should the doula not distract the woman from concentrating on coping with her labour, but the doula should also 'not *allow* her to be distracted' (my italics) (Klaus *et al.*, 1993: 139). The supportive role of the doula moves further in the direction of being differentiated from other carers' roles when Klaus and colleagues (1993: 7) refer to the likelihood of the woman being anxious that an outside person may take over or seek to assume control 'as many individuals providing labour assistance have traditionally done'. Thus, the doula is required to support relationships without interfering with them.

While it is unlikely to constitute a restriction on her activities, an interesting deficit in this area is the absence of research on the woman's experience of being cared for by a doula (Watkins, 1998). This leads to the suspicion that doula programmes do not warrant evaluation. Although this problem is addressed to some extent by Campero and colleagues' (1998) qualitative study, their work is of limited relevance to developed health care settings. Thus, although the doula's advocates draw heavily on RCT data, the experience of the individual woman does not feature. More typically in literature the mothers' words are filtered and interpreted by the doula (Klaus *et al.*, 1993: 18).

The emphasis by DONA (1999) on the non-medical and non-clinical role of the doula has been discussed earlier in this chapter (see 'Clinical functions' section). This point is pursued at some length, presumably to ensure that the message is driven home to potential clients, to potential doulas and to care providers who may feel threatened by this new arrival (Mainord, 1997; Abate, 2000, pers. comm.). This emphasis includes further mentions of the doula having been engaged separately by the family, thus making her clearly *not* a member of the hospital staff (DONA, 1999: 23). This situation may be changing, although the doula as hospital personnel is not yet accepted, as indicated by Simkin and Ancheta (2000):

> 'Some hospitals and health agencies have doulas on staff to help women as they are admitted, but most doulas contract privately with clients.'

The doula's relationship, in terms of status relative to the hospital personnel, is clearly spelt out. The terms used are reminiscent of hierarchies and verge on territoriality. Perhaps to reassure anxious care providers, the doula is compared with the person who is 'working in someone else's kitchen' (Klaus *et al.*, 1993: 22). This status gradient appears again when Klaus and colleagues warn that, in their highly medicalised system of childbirth, the doula should seek to avoid confrontation (Klaus, 1999: 139).

Thus, this perusal of what the doula does not do shows that she is expected to assume a relatively passive, facilitative role. In her performance of this role she should in no way challenge the status quo, although this possibility is clearly unlikely in view of her limited education and strictly subordinate position in the hierarchy. It soon becomes clear that the doula is in no position to challenge the medicalised system of childbearing within which she is expected to protect the interests of the woman. Least of all is the doula expected or able to challenge the staff who operate that system of childbirth – the medical practitioners. Thus, the ultimate restriction on her activity lies in the absolute veto on her exerting any form of threat to the medical order of childbearing.

The significance of the doula

Her advocates may argue that the advent of the doula on the childbearing scene heralds a new way of caring for the childbearing woman, particularly during labour. These arguments provide a stark contrast to the rationale advanced by Raphael (1973) and Sosa and colleagues (1980), who emphasised her historical existence and long standing anthropological credentials. The fervency of her advocates' enthusiasm for the doula verges on the evangelical, as is clearly reflected in the writing of Young (1998). Reference is made in inspirational jargon to the 'small group of far-seeing individuals ... who gathered to discuss the

concept and practice of support and companionship for women in labour'
(Young, 1998: 213). At the fourth conference, Young (1998: 213) recounts, she
found herself:

> 'swept up in the enthusiasm and commitment of a new generation of childbirth
> educators, nurses and other maternity caregivers who are supporting and
> energising each other in the development of this important new movement and
> profession.'

This manifesto finishes with a suitably anti-academic flourish which is tinged
with a flavour of other agendas, yet to be fully addressed:

> 'The scientific evidence of the benefits of this labour intervention cannot be
> questioned, however, and if hospitals want to improve the health and care of
> mothers and babies, and cut costs at the same time, implementing a doula
> program is in the best interests of everyone.'

(Young, 1998: 214)

This optimistic view of the future of the doula is also reflected in more mainstream publications (Olds *et al.*, 1996). Having reviewed the development of the
'labor support person', these authors observe that epidural analgesia is currently
'favoured'. When the epidural rates fall, 'as predicted' the doula will play a significant role in the less interventive forms of care in childbirth (Olds *et al.*, 1996:
299).

How has the doula phenomenon given rise to this frenzy of proselytising
among ordinarily level-headed practitioners? The religious analogy is appropriate. It may even be further and accurately extended to suggest that the doula
may be being perceived as some kind of saviour. On this occasion, however, it is
not souls which are to be saved from their fate.

The doula burst on to a maternity care scenario in the western hemisphere which
featured increasing intervention and increasing costs (see 'Finance' section in
Chapter 2). These developments have happened at the same time as and may be
associated with the move of childbirth from the woman's home to the institution
(Tew, 1995). It is possible that these factors may be linked with the increasing
tendency for medical personnel to be involved with maternity care in general and
with childbirth in particular. This tetrad is culminating in what is becoming known
as the 'caesarean epidemic' (Kitzinger, 1998; McCandlish, 1999; Flamm, 2000;
Porreco & Thorp, 1996) and is a cause of concern to many who are involved.

It becomes necessary to question the benefits of the interventive practice which
follows from medical involvement in childbearing and is associated, perhaps
coincidentally, with increasing caesarean rates and maternity costs. In spite of the
widespread use of a range of obstetric interventions, evidence of any improvement in morbidity and mortality rates is less than convincing (Flamm *et al.*, 1998;
WHO, 1985). It may be that in countries such as the USA, perinatal and infant
mortality rates are more comparable with those in third world countries than in
developed ones (Hanson, 2000b; Francome *et al.*, 1993). With the limited benefits

of interventive practice to the mother and baby, the spectre of unwarranted damage, which may be known as iatrogenesis, emerges (Robinson, 1999). While not improving the outcome for the mother and baby, interventions are increasing costs to insurance companies and other agencies which foot the health care bill.

Thus, the predicament appears to require action which will reverse these poor outcomes (Walton *et al.*, 1998; Fernandez *et al.*, 1999; Jabaaij & Meijer, 1996). This needs to take the form of a further intervention, because the process of medicalisation of birth is not amenable to being reversed (see section 'Medicalisation of maternity care' in Chapter 2). The reason for this is that medical power, which is sacrosanct, is dependent on medical intervention. The emergence of the support person in the findings of the Guatemalan studies (Sosa *et al.*, 1980; Klaus *et al.*, 1986), which were endorsed at almost the same time by the Dublin regime (O'Driscoll & Meagher, 1980), appeared as if in answer to the medical prayer (O'Regan, 1998). The doula was created and was welcomed fervently as the perfect solution to the predicament (Porreco & Thorp, 1996).

The doula was perceived as the solution for a number of reasons (Robinson, 1999). First, the problematic situation relates to maternity costs (Scott *et al.*, 1999) and the doula is a low cost answer, due to being untrained or minimally trained, with no career path or aspirations (Klaus *et al.*, 1993: 135) and female. Second, she is the solution because the problems are medically generated and the doula exerts no threat to medical practitioners, as she is relatively lacking in expert knowledge. Third, she offers no challenge to medical power because she is low status in the organisational hierarchy and female. Fourth, as an ideal solution she does not threaten accepted medical practice or the status quo, because she may be slotted into the existing system of maternity care. Finally, the acceptance of the doula actually enhances medical status through endorsing the research credentials of her medical advocates. This is because her effectiveness has been scientifically established by a series of RCTs. Additionally, for those who continue to doubt the value of research evidence, the experience of the Dublin regime supports her effect on the caesarean rate, a major component of the predicament (Klaus & Kennell, 1997). The extent of the anticipated reduction in health care costs associated with the employment of a doula is large; it has been estimated at about $3,500 per woman's labour (Klaus *et al.*, 1993: 31).

In this way, the doula not only permits the continuation of the medicalisation of childbearing, but she also limits any iatrogenic effects (Robinson, 1999) or other costs (Klaus *et al.*, 1993: 31), such as further increases in the caesarean rate. This assumption is relatively safe because her presence in even less salubrious childbearing conditions has been shown by RCTs to be beneficial. It is with these developments as the background that the findings of a systematic review are used to recommend:

'adoption of hospital policies encouraging the presence of experienced lay women, including female relatives.'

(Hodnett, 2000c: 7)

Implications for other maternity personnel

The analysis of the beneficial effects of the introduction of the doula for our medical colleagues has been applied to those situations where medicalised maternity care is *de rigueur*. It may be safe to assume that this applies to the majority of westernised health care environments. There is, however, another factor which needs to be taken into account when seeking to understand this conundrum. As two of the RCT research teams (Madi *et al.*, 1999; Campero *et al.*, 1998) explain, in their countries, Botswana and Mexico respectively, a traditionally supportive form of care had been usurped by medicalisation. The iatrogenic effects of these developments were of such magnitude that it needed a specific support person to be introduced via the RCTs in order to 'undo' the damage and facilitate the physiological processes in the labouring woman.

In other countries the maternity situation may be different again. It is necessary to question the relevance of the RCTs to developed countries with an ongoing tradition of supportive midwifery care. As I have indicated, in such settings the midwife's ideal role is fundamentally similar to that of the doula (Siddiqui, 1999). It may be that the process of medicalisation there may be less complete than in Botswana and in Mexico. The question of whether the midwife in such settings is permitted to practise holistically and to provide effective support for the woman in labour still needs to be asked.

The factors which impede such a complete practice of supportive midwifery, though quantitatively different, may still bear comparison. Thus, midwifery practice in countries such as the UK may still be limited by organisational factors. These may include funds being allocated inappropriately. The result is that the midwife is prevented, due to a lack of suitable staff (Scott *et al.*, 1999), from providing the supportive care which she knows to be necessary and is well able and keen to provide. Additionally, the midwife's ability to offer effective support may be further limited by the protocols within which she is required to practise. These are medically dominated and effectively reduce her practice to that of an obstetric nurse (Walker, 1976). Whether these organisational changes have been introduced in spite of her, or whether they have been facilitated by the passive acquiescence of the midwife, is not easy to assess. Thus, the issue which needs to be considered is that, while midwifery care in the UK may not be the ideal form of care, it constitutes a base on which to build. This is preferable to abandoning the existing pattern of care in order to introduce another which has been researched only in very different settings (Hodnett, 2000c).

Conclusion

The point has been made that the doula has been presented as the way of meeting the needs of the childbearing woman. I have argued that this is a misrepresentation of the facts; the doula is nothing more than a medical answer to the needs of the medical practitioner and the predicament which he has created in the course of the medicalisation of maternity care in general and childbirth in particular. Analogies featuring the rearrangement of deck chairs on sinking ships and the use of a sticking plaster to control haemorrhage leap to mind. The doula serves no function other than to permit the continuing escalation of the medicalisation of childbirth.

The introduction of this new support person is addressed by Odent (1996) in his critical appraisal of the benefits or otherwise of support in labour. Odent emphasises the internality of the woman's focus in labour. He emphasises that the woman is ideally suited to giving birth, as long as the physiological, including endocrinological and emotional, processes are permitted to proceed unhindered. Any hindrance may be in the form of questioning the woman or altering her environment in such a way that her focus is redirected away from herself.

The argument being advanced by Odent may be summarised in terms of 'If it ain't broke don't fix it' and is presented at two levels. The first, which I have mentioned already, relates to the processes of labour in the individual woman. The second level relates to the organisation of maternity care in seeking to provide the appropriate environment in which labour is able to proceed unhindered. This environment includes the wide range of physical and emotional aspects which I discussed in Chapter 5. At this second level, Odent (1996: 51) includes the midwife as a crucial component of the facilitative environment:

> 'Where there are many midwives and a small number of well trained obstetricians ... the birth outcomes are much better.'

Thus, irrespective of the questions hanging over the introduction of the doula in health care systems which no longer feature the midwife, in those systems that include a midwife the doula is superfluous. The woman in labour clearly does not need to be assisted by this additional import from an alien childbearing culture.

Chapter 7
Support for the carer

Up to this point in this book the focus has been on the support available to the childbearing woman. I have addressed the need for and provision of support, as well as critically analysing the source of that support. In this chapter, though, I would like to redirect our attention on to the needs of the person who provides that support. I shall consider whether and to what extent she in turn is appropriately supported.

Concerns about high levels of student nurse attrition served as the trigger to initiate the research project which eventually became a classic study of personnel support among hospital staff (Revans, 1964). This study built on Menzies' (1960) equally well-known and respected research. She had shown how the organisation of nursing activities acts as a potentially counterproductive defence against unacknowledged anxiety. Revans also showed the crucial nature of the practices used to cope with anxiety and the practices which serve to aggravate it. That the terms 'stress' and 'anxiety' may be used interchangeably is evident in the work of Niven (1992), making the discussion in Chapter 1 relevant here. The association between stress/anxiety and health problems (section 'Support and health' in Chapter 1) has long been well-established (Cherniss, 1980). A then novel concept which emerged from Revans' (1964) study, and which has subsequently been repeatedly endorsed (Stoter, 1997: 3), is the direct and positive correlation between the limited support of personnel and their reduced ability to provide caring support for clients and patients. For this reason, if for no other, it is essential to contemplate whether and how personnel are cared for and whether and how they care for each other.

In this chapter I use the relevant research to contemplate, first, the role of social support for workers and employees in general. Next, I adjust the focus to look at the work relating to our nursing cousins and certain others and the extent to which it is relevant to the midwife. The phenomenon which has become known as 'burnout' gradually emerges and becomes increasingly significant in the context of midwifery. I next consider the rather limited research interest in the support provided for the midwife herself. While research in this area is lacking, the not unrelated subject of midwifery supervision has benefited from more research attention and this is the next topic to be addressed. Finally, in order to illustrate some of the issues to which reference has been made, I consider the significance of support as it emerged in a study of the midwife's experience of the death of a mother in her care (Mander, 1999a, b).

Staff support in general

Because this chapter focuses on the midwife in her professional capacity and because much of the literature on support uses the work situation as its context, it is in the general workplace that this analysis of the subject will begin. It may be, due to a large majority of midwives being women and due to much of this research having been undertaken in male-dominated settings, that this analysis is less than totally realistic. Whether this is the case will become clearer as this examination of the subject progresses and the focus on the midwife becomes more precise.

As with so many phenomena, when its benefits were first suspected social support was widely regarded as a panacea, in that it was thought to be at least capable of solving a wide range of, if not all, personal difficulties. Etzion (1984) recounts the initial identification of the moderating or buffering effects of social support on stress and strain. The variables which tend to be responsible for stress in employees include bureaucratic pressures and a lack of feedback, autonomy and appreciation. Etzion goes on to quote House to suggest that the form of support which may reduce such stresses comprises 'an interpersonal transaction involving one or more of the following features: emotional concern, instrumental aid, information and appraisal' (House, 1981).

One of the constructs which has been linked with social support and which may also serve to reduce occupational stress is control. Baker and colleagues (1996) investigated the widespread assumption that it is a combination of high work demands and low worker control which leads to poor health outcomes. These researchers sought to disentangle the relationship between support and control in the reduction of occupational stress. The research was undertaken in an industrial setting, referred to as 'a plant', in the USA. The proportion of male employees was large, but that may actually make the findings relating to support more relevant here rather than less. A number of instruments were used to measure support, including two to measure co-worker social support in the form of affective support and instrumental support with work-related problems. Additionally there were two instruments to measure supervisor support in the form of affective and instrumental supervisorial support.

Baker and colleagues found that the generally beneficial effects of control and involvement were moderated by organisational aspects, suggesting the complexity of the phenomena. Although similarly generally beneficial, the effects of social support were found to be dependent on other variables. The source of that support, whether peer or supervisor, and its nature, whether affective or instrumental, were found to be crucial. It was also found that any increase in support, whether affective or instrumental, from a supervisor was more than likely to be associated with decreased negative job feelings, that is, greater satisfaction.

The significance of Baker and colleagues' sample comprising a largely male workforce deserves attention. The effects of gender on social support were highlighted by Etzion as early as 1984 when she showed the different moderating influences on stress in women and men. She demonstrated that for women work stress is buffered by social support from both relatives and friends. For men, however, this moderation is by work support by supervisors and fellow workers. Etzion goes on to warn that this form of buffering applies more to work stress than to the potentially more intimate aspects of life stress. The difference in the source of buffering or support, she maintains, relates to the location of the individual's 'central life interest' (Etzion, 1984: 621), resulting in more work-oriented support for men. As well as such gendered differences, Etzion emphasises the need to take into account ethnic and cultural influences on support mechanisms. It may be that changing patterns of work among women and men require that these findings and the assumptions to which they are related need to be re-examined.

This material on support in manufacturing industry provides a general background to the present state of knowledge. The need for support for staff working in a therapeutic environment, addressed by Sudbery and Bradley (1996), demonstrates further issues relevant to support in the maternity setting. At the risk of stating the obvious, they point out the fundamental nature of genuinely open human engagement on the effectiveness of any helping relationship. Having emphasised the benefits of engagement, these authors suggest the possibility that it may be facilitated, in the form of increased empathy, through 'counter-transference'. This concept comprises reflexive responses by the care provider, which lead to a 'virtuous spiral'. Unfortunately, there is also the risk that these responses may be counterproductive. Negative outcomes may arise from the carer's previous unhappy experience or from complementary emotional processes, such as unrelieved stress. Clearly such countertransference would limit the effectiveness of any help being offered, while at the same time aggravating the emotional difficulty of the carer. In this situation it would be a vicious cycle which would develop due to the absence of good support for staff.

Sudbery and Bradley (1996) move on to discuss the degree of formality of staff support. Employee Assistance Programmes (EAPs) are a North American import, which originally addressed only specific areas such as drug or alcohol problems. Their wider application, though, has been shown to reduce staff sickness and absence rates. Inevitably, such formalised schemes raise a multiplicity of ethical problems, such as who benefits from EAPs. Additionally, concerns about confidentiality may reduce their use, as attendance may be perceived as constituting evidence of unsuitability for employment. Such concerns become more acute in the less than ideal situations where the supporter is also the line manager. Clearly, if there is a line relationship the support must be confidential, and rigorously separated from appraisal procedures. It may be that such support is better provided as an extended form of the role of the occupational health department. The issue of the source of support for managers and supervisors, however, remains uncertain. The concerns voiced about EAPs apply no less to the better known Staff Support Groups (Lederberg, 1998).

The organisation of support in caring environments is not the only hurdle which needs to be overcome among both staff and managers. Unhelpful attitudes which regard any form of help as a self indulgent luxury needed only by wimps, may still exist. Thus, Sudbery and Bradley (1996) plead for a change in the culture of caring. This should result in the removal of any stigma and make care for the fellow worker as routine or 'natural' as care for the client.

There are certain other occupational groups, who may not be regarded as carers but who are relevant here. These include the firefighters, paramedics and other emergency personnel who, because of their unusual work patterns and the hazards inherent in their work, highlight certain important aspects of occupational support (Beaton *et al.*, 1997). Their long shifts, less than sociable hours of work and periods of inaction interspersed with hectic and challenging activity increase the likelihood of strong within-group social support. There is always the possibility, though, of such networks acting as double edged swords. Because of the tendency of these workers to socialise together, the differentiation between work and non-work support is not always clear. In a comparison of home and work support, the researchers found that home social support is effective in providing protection from post traumatic stress disorder. It was found, though, that support at work has a stronger effect, which may be due to its 'relevancy' and timeliness. Yet again, the primacy of work-related social support in a predominantly male group becomes apparent.

Nurses' support

Because their working lives share certain features and because many midwives possess both a nursing qualification and nursing experience, it is appropriate to consider here the literature on social support for nurses. In spite of the many differences between these two occupational groups, this 'disclaimer' may not be entirely necessary in view of the general consistency in the literature on general employees, nurses and midwives.

With the spectre of burnout never very far away and considering the institutional, staff and individual strategies, Burr (1996) examines the support needed for and offered to nurses working with people with HIV/AIDS. The first line of approach is at an institutional level; the focus, however, should be on the individual by helping her to, for example, implement a self/peer care programme and to develop a more appropriately internal locus of control. Institutional recognition of the stressful nature of the nurse's work is recommended in the form of time out after a particularly difficult encounter or for 'mental health days'. Another example of this recognition might be encouraging the nurse to attend the funeral of someone who had been a client.

Members of staff may be encouraged to offer peer support in the form of mentoring by more experienced colleagues. Group support may be facilitated, although careful planning is necessary with regard to the ground rules relating to confidentiality and composition of the group. On an individual basis, the role of family and friends is seen as unfailingly helpful. Similarly, a stress reduction activity may be chosen by each individual nurse because it is effective for her. The role of both humour and spirituality are recognised for their benefits in terms of physiological and psychological as well as group functioning.

Like Baker and colleagues (1996), Munro *et al.* (1998) examined occupational stress in relation to how the tension between control and demand may be ameliorated by social support. The important differences between these studies are that the first sampled a largely male work force in an American factory, whereas the second sampled a predominantly female group of psychiatric nurses in Australia. Many of the findings of these two studies, however, are comparable. Munro and colleagues identified the likelihood of the demands of a situation being moderated by the supportiveness of that situation. Thus, a job with high demands was not necessarily stressful if it was accompanied by a high level of support from fellow workers.

This research by Munro and colleagues may also be compared with that by Beaton *et al.* (1997) on firefighters and paramedics. Both groups of researchers sought to compare support at work with non-work support to assess which is the more effective. Munro's findings differed crucially in that non-work support was found to be more significant than work support. Whether this was associated with the different gender of the samples, in support of Etzion's (1984) observation, may only be surmised. The Australian study like so many others firmly endorsed the protective nature of social support against a range of stress-related health problems. These researchers, however, were able to extend this protection beyond the reality of support, as they found that the perception of being supported is also associated with being healthier and more satisfied.

The satisfactions and stresses of one particular area of nursing (stoma care) were investigated by Hingley and Marks (1991) using a Nurse Stress Index and stress diaries. These researchers identified the immense job satisfaction experienced by this group of nurses, but also found a number of factors giving rise to stress. Factors which engendered organisational stress included uncertainty about the nurse's role and also relationships with the team and other personnel. The need for the over-worked stoma nurse to travel between sites and clinical areas served to aggravate stress which was compounded by feelings of being isolated and lacking managerial support. Because of insufficient time at work these nurses experienced an overspill of the less desirable aspects of work, such as taking administrative tasks home.

Because it has been suggested that the nurse's stress is related to the specialist area of her work, an attempt was made to study nurses in different clinical settings (Hillhouse & Adler, 1997). The social support of colleagues was again found to be an important resource in all settings. These researchers found that this operates by promoting a sense of competence, which leads to self-efficacy, which in turn generates increased self-esteem. The main stressors identified among the 260 respondents include 'death and suffering', 'conflict with other nurses' and 'uncertainty and/or lack of preparation'. The nurses observed that although these stressors are most significant, they are not as damaging to the individual nurse as 'conflict with physicians'.

The researchers found that effective support strengthens relationships within the ward unit and serves to buffer the effects of interpersonal stressors. Lack of support, on the other hand, aggravates conflict and emotional and physical strain. A negative correlation was found between social support and levels of burnout. Thus, levels of burnout were found to be high in ward units where social support was low. The effects of poor interpersonal relations, especially with physicians, were a serious concern. It was found that *intra*professional conflict was less threatening. The authors suggest that medical power and status increase the significance of *inter*professional conflict, escalating the threat and the stress and giving rise to greater symptomatology.

Burnout

When thinking about stress in helping professions such as nursing and midwifery, the spectre of burnout is never too far away (Burr, 1996; Hillhouse & Adler,1997; Matrunola, 1996). Unfortunately it is a term, like 'stress', which tends to attract considerable attention from those with little understanding of its meaning. As Hawkins and Shohet (1989: 20) observe:

> '[Burnout] has become the helping professions' equivalent to what the British army called "shell shock" or the Americans "battle fatigue"; what our parents' generation called "nerves" and the present generation "depression". They become catch-all phrases that signify not coping.'

For these reasons, 'burnout' may have become discredited. It is, therefore, necessary to consider what this term actually means before examining its significance for the helping professionals in general and for the midwife in particular.

The meaning of burnout

As shown by the quotation above, the difficulty which some people may encounter when they face challenging situations has long been recognised. Our understanding of stress and its causes and effects increased exponentially with the ground-breaking work of Selye (1956). That those who provide care are far from immune soon became apparent. The possibility of burnout among caring professionals was attributed to too-high expectations of their own ability and invulnerability, perhaps in a form of professional arrogance (Edelwich & Brodsky, 1980). This implicit criticism is endorsed by an early definition of burnout: 'To fail, wear out, or become exhausted by making excessive demands on their energy, strength or resources' (Cherniss, 1980: 16).

That burnout is a long term condition, as opposed to an acute one, is emphasised by Etzion (1984). This chronicity is endorsed by Hillhouse and Adler (1997) who differentiate burnout from stress in terms of the former being a process rather than an incident or event. Burnout is a maladaptive form of psychological accommodation. It develops initially as a psychological process to produce outward affective and physical symptoms, which are associated with the worker's negative experience of job strain.

Much of the research on burnout has used the instrument devised by Maslach (the MBI or Maslach Burnout Inventory), whose definition distinguishes the component parts of this phenomenon (Maslach, 1981):

'A syndrome of emotional exhaustion, depersonalisation and reduced personal accomplishment.'

These three aspects of burnout may be regarded as sequential phases in the development of burnout (Maslach, 1976; Burnard, 1991).

Emotional exhaustion is associated with the carer feeling that she has little left to give to others, perhaps due to 'having given her all'. This interpretation resonates with the views mentioned above (Edelwich & Brodsky, 1980) of the health carer being the provider and the client the recipient. This view may be contrasted with the healthier 'partnership' relationship which is often advocated. This form of fatigue leads to the carer becoming increasingly disengaged or detached.

Depersonalisation is characterised by the carer's detachment leading to alienation from both clients or patients and colleagues. Negative feelings about those with whom she works are prevalent to the extent that avoidance tactics may be employed, such as becoming immersed in mind numbing administrative tasks.

Reduced personal accomplishment may be the real result of these avoidance tactics or may be due to difficulty in assessing actual work performance both past and present. This disillusionment may lead to a career change or the person persevering against what are perceived as the odds.

Midwives and burnout

It may be because maternity is ordinarily perceived as a happy area in which to work that the literature on burnout among midwives has been, until recently, relatively scanty. An exception to this is the study by Beaver *et al.* (1986) which involved the application of the MBI to 98 USA educated and employed certified nurse-midwives (CNMs). The findings revealed that the majority of the respondents reported low levels of burnout on all six MBI dimensions. However, high levels of burnout, ranging from 8.2% to 21.4% for each of the six MBI dimensions, were found. Burnout was found to be more likely to occur in CNMs who:

(1) Were younger
(2) Had more children
(3) Were relatively newly employed in large services serving a high proportion of low socio-economic class families
(4) Lacked collegial and consumer support.

The relevance of this study to the present discussion, though, is uncertain in view of the low response rate and the precarious position of American nurse-midwifery in 1982 when the data were collected.

Some of the more recent literature may have been influenced by burnout's 'bad press', as it may comprise little more than a plea to retain the status quo (such as Barber, 1998). The corollary of this abuse of the term has resulted in its avoidance by other midwives, where the concept is clearly relevant. An example of its unmentioned relevance is in a clinical setting where burnout would be a distinct occupational hazard; this is a wing in a maternity unit which is specifically designated to meet the needs of parents who are experiencing some form of loss in childbearing (Foster, 1996). In this wing the maintenance of healthy therapeutic relationships between staff and clients and among staff is fostered by using specific strategies, including:

(1) Promotion of team spirit
(2) Formal staff counselling training
(3) Management support
(4) Counselling for the counsellors (supervision).

This account, unfortunately, becomes prescriptive rather than descriptive for strategies 2 and 4, suggesting that these are aims and are not yet achieved. Some of the likely reasons for the non-achievement of these aims feature in the explanation by Bakker and colleagues of the factors aggravating the occurrence of burnout. These factors include 'insufficient training, a shortage of personnel or a lack of support from colleagues and superiors' (Bakker *et al.*, 1996: 176).

Another research project in which the term 'burnout' seems to have been strenuously avoided was undertaken in Northern Ireland (Mackin & Sinclair, 1998). The sample comprised 43 labour ward midwives and the assessment tools were the General Health Questionnaire (version 12) and a specially designed questionnaire. The researchers identified that a number of factors were thought to aggravate the midwife's stress. A major factor is the lack of time to complete the work which the midwife considers necessary. Interestingly, other people in the labour ward were mainly to blame for causing unnecessary stress. This criticism applied to the 'auxiliary', to the women's visitors and equally to midwifery and medical staff. In general terms, the midwife's external locus of control appears to be responsible for her morbidly high stress levels.

The research by Bakker and colleagues (1996) on burnout among midwives is important because it, unusually, recognises that there may be negative aspects to the Dutch system of maternity care. This study is probably unique because the system is almost invariably praised to the point of being recommended as a model for replication (Mander,1995). It may even be that certain aspects of Dutch maternity care are already being replicated in the UK system and that Bakker and colleagues' study may serve as a timely warning of the UK midwife's future health status.

This Dutch study focused on 200 community midwives and their practice. Data were collected through, first, detailed diaries, second, a questionnaire on practice and personal characteristics and, third, a questionnaire on burnout, coping and social support. These researchers found that the midwife's degree of depersonalisation correlates positively with the size of the group practice within which she works, rather than with the level of urbanisation of her working environment (Bakker *et al.*, 1996: 180). They also found that a higher proportion of home births is associated with a lower risk of burnout; the researchers suggest that this finding is likely to be mediated by greater job satisfaction. The corollary of this observation is that a high proportion of short stay hospital births correlates with more profound emotional tension.

Bakker and colleagues go on to suggest a remedy by observing the significance of personal resources, such as social support and coping style, in ameliorating the process of burnout. They recommend educational modifications in order to reduce the potentially harmful effects of working as a midwife in the Netherlands. Their midwifery educational programmes may need to be amended to include sessions on strategies to facilitate both peer support and personal coping.

Burnout was also a prominent finding in a recent research project in England (Sandall, 1997, 1998, 1999). Sandall sought to study the impact on the midwife's work and personal life of recent developments in the organisation of midwifery care. These developments are often known by the title of the English government department publication *Changing Childbirth* (Chapter 4; DoH, 1993). Sandall's research involved a multiplicity of methods. First were interviews and observations at sites which demonstrated the innovative forms of midwifery care (stage 1). This stage investigated the meaning which the midwife attaches to her work and how she integrates the various aspects of her life.

Then followed stage 2, which comprised a regionally stratified random postal survey of 5% of the members of the Royal College of Midwives in England. The survey questions were chosen on the basis of the findings of stage 1 and focused on work, family circumstances and the measurement of stress. The data collection instruments included the General Health Questionnaire (version 12) and an adaptation of the MBI (see the previous section). Of the1166 questionnaires distributed 800 were returned completed, giving a response rate of 69%. Comparisons made included the stressful and the satisfying aspects of midwifery work, and comparison of midwifery practice in the community and in the hospital.

The stage 1 interviews and observations were with midwives at three sites where continuity of care differs. Autonomy, social support and meaningfulness of relationships with women proved to be significant themes. All of the midwives valued collegial social support as a stress reducer, but when it was lacking this lack itself became a major source of stress. The midwife's domestic support or lack of it was found to have similar effects. The presence of children may be perceived as either a stressor or as a buffer against stress, but Sandall found that children served to protect the midwife from overcommitment to her work. Similarly, children may have prevented the midwife from becoming involved in certain over-taxing practice arrangements. Approximately one fifth of the midwives claimed to be burned-out in association with poor colleague support, fragmented client contact, too heavy a workload, too high expectations, or lack of domestic emotional/social support. On the other hand the midwives with high levels of personal accomplishment reported assertive and realistic relationships. Examples of satisfactory relationships included those with colleagues, women and 'family'. Collegial work support, domestic emotional/social support and appropriate non-work time and non-work activities also featured as contributing healthily.

On the basis of the MBI it was found that 26% of the midwives had high emotional exhaustion scores, but high personal accomplishment scores were also identified. Factors relating to the midwife's working hours were the main predictor of burnout. Sandall found that midwives who were working for more than 37.5 hours per week showed higher burnout scores (22.5%) than their colleagues who worked under 20 hours per week (18%). This finding suggests that Etzion's (1984) observation may be accurate, as these midwives are likely to be working reduced hours because of their family commitments and Etzion suggested that family ties are associated with lower levels of stress.

In terms of the conditions under which these midwives worked, certain NHS organisational structures were more stressful, especially when applied to midwifery practice. Burnout was found to be highest among hospital team midwives and lowest among traditional community midwives who were 'GP attached'. Sandall suggests that the hospital team midwives had the least control over their working lives. This may be linked with the importance of relationships with medical personnel as found among midwives and nurses (Mackin & Sinclair, 1998; Hillhouse & Adler, 1997).

On the basis of these findings Sandall seeks to redefine burnout in terms of disillusionment, rather than the usual three characteristics mentioned in the previous section (Maslach, 1976). She also suggests that the factors associated with burnout, which she refers to as 'predictors', should be taken into account when planning further developments in the organisation of midwifery practice. She does, however, recommend that further longitudinal studies are necessary to ascertain the predictive value of the predictors to which she refers.

Thus, it is apparent that the experience of burnout, although traditionally thought to be less likely among midwives than among other groups of employees, may be aggravated by certain developments which have been introduced with the intention of benefiting both the woman and her carer. In the same way as burnout among midwives is now the subject of more, and more appropriate, research attention, one of the possible remedies, supervision, is now also receiving the research attention which it deserves.

Supervision

As a helping intervention, supervision is in a state of flux. Although it is a system which has been part of English midwifery since 1902 (Jenkins, 1995), it originally comprised a rigid form of control unknown to any other occupational group or profession. Since that time the same term has been adopted by other helping professions and has become known as 'clinical supervision' among our nursing cousins. Simultaneously midwifery supervision has evolved in a subtly different direction. These developments have given rise to widespread confusion about the meaning of the term 'supervision' and its nature (Deery & Corby, 1996).

Clinical supervision

Psychotherapy, social work and counselling are the disciplines in which clinical supervision has been long established. Areas of nursing with strong links with these disciplines, such as mental health nursing, were the first to make use of it. Its adoption, though, may be due to the similar challenges of the relationships fundamental to the work rather than to a direct transfer (Playle & Mullarkey, 1998). The purpose of clinical supervision has been explained in a number of ways. Examples are to increase the carer's effectiveness, to improve account-ability and efficiency, to ensure the carer's compliance to unit policies or to create a consultancy role to support and facilitate the development of the carer (Hawkins & Shohet, 1989). The last interpretation is the one which currently predominates in nursing, summarised by Butterworth and Faugier (1992: 238) as 'to grow emotionally and professionally'.

Supervision of the midwife

Although the origins of midwifery supervision are clearly different, the underlying rationale may be less so. Clinical supervision is primarily 'to protect clients' (Playle & Mullarkey, 1998: 560), whereas midwifery supervision is intended 'to protect the public' (NBS, 1999). Attempts to achieve this aim may have led to certain notorious 'cases' in the past which may have brought the system of midwifery supervision into disrepute (Beech, 1993). These cases have involved fraught relationships between supervisors and a certain group of midwives. This parti-cularly vulnerable group of midwives is known as 'independent midwives' because their practice is largely outside the UK National Health Service (Isherwood, 1989).

The role of the supervisor of midwives is determined by the Midwives Rules (UKCC, 1999). She is the person to whom is delegated the role of ensuring that the midwife reaches and maintains a satisfactory level of competence. The supervisor relates to the midwife within geographical and/or functional boundaries. The role of the supervisor involves certain potentially conflicting aspects which may have resulted in the difficult and possibly notorious situations referred to. This difficult role consists of offering support by being a 'guide, counsellor and friend' to the midwife over whom the supervisor also happens to have the power to suspend from duty and perhaps from practice (Isherwood, 1988).

While the focus on the client's benefit from midwifery supervision is overwhelming in one statutory body's documentation, little reference is made to the supportive aspects of this role. Such reference is limited merely to 'supporting midwives at a time of major change' (NBS, 1999) and 'the facilitative and supportive role' of the supervisor (NBS, undated). In spite of this disconcerting neglect of the peer support element inherent in supervision by one statutory body, midwife authors perceive the supervisor as having the potential to provide support in the following ways:

- Practice development
- Responding to dubiously appropriate requests
- Investigating allegations
- Recognising poor practice
- In the event of litigation   (Johnson, 1996: 97)

- Adapting to new working arrangements
- Fulfilling educational needs
- Setting/auditing clinical standards
- Maintaining inter-professional relationships   (Warwick, 1996: 105)

- Taking concerns seriously
- Solving organisational problems   (Shennan, 1996: 167)

Additionally, an important research project (Stapleton *et al.*, 1998) has further served to redress the imbalance between the emphasis on supervisor as 'watchdog' or 'friend' (Isherwood, 1988). This project, commissioned by the English National Board and the UKCC, comprised, first of all, an audit of supervisors and arrangements for supervision. The second, qualitative, part of the project involved in-depth interviews and focus groups with midwives, with supervisors and with users of the midwifery services. Following the collection of these data, midwives provided their personal constructs which allowed a value grid to be drawn up. The data were collected at five contrasting sites in England. The sixth 'site' comprised midwives whose practice was outside the mainstream NHS system of maternity care.

Power relationships

The researchers were able to draw a number of conclusions relating to the midwife's working environment and particularly to the balance of power within that environment. The general picture which emerges is to some extent reminiscent of the maladaptive strategies to cope with anxiety which were identified more than 30 years ago among our nursing cousins (Menzies, 1960). These defence mechanisms, which have been identified by others' research, in midwifery include stereotyping and blaming clients and the inverse care law (Stapleton *et al.*, 1998: 32).

The social environment within which midwives work, rather than featuring supportive, nurturing peer relationships, is characterised by the phenomenon which has been entitled 'horizontal violence' (Friere, 1972). This phenomenon typically comprises a relatively weak group sharing an environment, such as the workplace, with another group which is stronger. Stapleton and colleagues explicitly identify this dominant group as our medical colleagues (Stapleton *et al.*, 1998: 21). The weaker group is unable to actively and constructively seek to redress its disadvantaged status. The members of the weaker group therefore gain satisfaction, in the form of some semblance of power, through negative behaviours towards each other. With embarrassing honesty Leap (1997: 689) recounts the forms which such behaviours may take among her midwifery colleagues in Australia:

'... overt and covert non-physical hostility, such as sabotage, infighting, scapegoating, backstabbing and negative criticism. The failure to respect privacy or keep confidences, non-verbal innuendo, undermining, lack of openness, unwillingness to help out and lack of support...'

Clearly a response in the form of horizontal violence has the potential to be counterproductive. In this way it may have the effect of further weakening the group's already subservient position.

Collegial support

As may happen in any number of childbearing situations (Mander, 1992), the midwives in Stapleton and colleagues' (1998) study identify strongly with the women for whom they provide care. This applies no less to the midwife's need for psychosocial support from her colleagues. In terms of the provision of support, these researchers show the painfully stark contrast between the support which midwives feel they should, and presumably do, provide for childbearing women, and the support which they make available to each other. It may be assumed that this extension of such supportive behaviour to colleagues may be a commonplace which is taken for granted. This important and authoritative research project, however, suggests that this is far from the case:

'... there was a painful contradiction between their need for support, and the fact that the culture of midwifery could not acknowledge, nor provide for that need.'

(Stapleton *et al.*, 1998: 142)

Role models

Stapleton and colleagues draw attention to the problems created by the lack of positive role models for and among midwives. Not surprisingly, in a research report on supervision this applies particularly to the supervisor of midwives. It is argued that the supervisor should be able to act as a positive role model in the provision of peer support. Hence, the midwives whom she supervises would be able to emulate her caring approach to her colleagues.

What emerges from this research, though, is that the supervisor is likely to find that she lacks adequate support from *her* supervisor. Thus, the support which she is able to offer is severely limited, as is her effectiveness as a role model. For this reason, the midwife's supervisor is prevented from demonstrating even that she is good at looking after herself. Effectively the tables are turned from the ideal role model arrangement to the extent that the 'midwives frequently expressed sympathy and concern for [the supervisors]' (Stapleton *et al.*, 1998: 143).

Culture

The social environment of the midwife's workplace comprises a powerfully prevailing culture, which influences a wide range of the midwives' feelings about and reactions to midwifery (Kirkham, 1999, 2000). The effect of the culture of service and sacrifice results in the midwife feeling guilty and 'selfish' that she should be experiencing such feelings as needing support. The culture also exerts pressure on the individual midwife to conform to the status quo, which results in her dutiful, if sorrowful, adherence to the established norm and effectively prevents her from breaking ranks.

Good practice

The crucial role of both midwifery supervision and the supervisor of midwives is strongly endorsed by the study by Stapleton and colleagues (1998). These researchers found that, while these roles have the potential to benefit both the midwife and her practice on a long term basis, there is also the potential for them to exert the reverse effect. That supervision may work well emerges in some examples of good practice. These examples were reported by midwives who found that their experience of enjoying 'empowering' supervision (Stapleton *et al.*, 1998: 148) served to facilitate a change in their practice in the direction of becoming more confident and assertive. Supervision, when it takes this form, is likely to be challenging in a positive sense, requiring the midwife to justify her practice both intellectually and emotionally.

A research project

Midwives' support for each other emerged as a major theme in a recent research project on the midwife facing one particularly challenging clinical situation. These findings illustrate certain important issues relating to formal and informal systems of support for the midwife. It is helpful to look closely at this research in order to emphasise, and also to make comparisons with, other researchers' findings.

Although it may not be part of one's own personal experience, many will know or know of a midwife whose experience of the death of a mother in her care destroyed her career and, possibly, her. Some may, like me, have been in a position to witness the reactions of those midwives who, although not directly involved, were affected by the death. The effect on each individual midwife is disconcerting, but it has been my observation that the effect on the group of midwives is neither common, shared nor uniform. It was my impression that each midwife was dealing individually with her own anxieties and seeking to exorcise her own ghosts.

My personal observations have shown me, however, that there are some reactions which are shared. These relate mainly to the dead woman's family. Invariably the baby inspires pity, through being deprived of the loving care that is unique to motherhood. Inevitably this pity is tinged with anxiety about how the 'child' will cope when she becomes a parent, with no experience of mothering on which to base her own childcare. To a marginally lesser extent the father also inspires pity. This tends to be moderated, though, by incredulity that this man's reaction to his bereavement should be somewhat less obvious than would be expected if a woman were to be bereaved of her life-partner. Concern for the father may also be constrained by anxiety concerning the possibility of litigation.

The person who, I have observed, is not the object of pity, sympathy or any other fellow-feeling by those who are uninvolved is the midwife who was responsible for the woman's care at the time. This midwife's practice may be scrutinised scathingly, though not to her face. Any previous problems and errors are likely to be resurrected and dissected. There is invariably a tendency to draw conclusions along the lines of 'an accident waiting to happen'. Such covert criticism is thinly disguised in an attempt to maintain a 'normal' working atmosphere. This charade is hard work for all involved, especially for the midwife at the centre of the 'case', who is concurrently dealing with statements, investigations, uncertain outcomes as well as the gamut of emotions.

Thus, a research project was planned on the basis of these observations and impressions and the scanty literature which has been published (Mander, 1999a). The research project sought answers to the following questions:

(1) How is the midwife affected by the experience of caring for a mother who dies?
(2) After a mother for whom she has cared has died, what interventions does the midwife identify as either helpful or unhelpful to her?
(3) Does the distant possibility of death influence the practice of a midwife caring for a mother who is experiencing an uncomplicated pregnancy or childbirth or post natal period? If so, in what way does this influence operate?

The relevance of this research to the present discussion on stress and burnout may be questioned, particularly in view of the death of a mother usually being a relatively acute episode. It may be, though, that the three aspects of burnout mentioned earlier in this chapter in the section 'The meaning of burnout', become more relevant when the potentially long term effects of this experience on the midwife, her relationships and her practice are taken into account.

In view of the limited literature available on the midwife's experience of caring for a mother who dies, it was clear that qualitative methods would be the more suitable approach. Data were collected mainly through semi-structured telephone interviews with midwives who had had this experience. To answer the third question (above) a sample of midwives without this experience ('non-experienced midwives') would also be sought. Because of the sensitivity of the topic the sample could comprise only volunteers. The small number of anticipated respondents was unlikely to be a problem, as qualitative methods seek to obtain deeper rather than broader data. Volunteers were to be recruited through one of the more popular midwifery publications (Mander, 1999a).

Each of the informants gave permission for the interview to be taped. It was later transcribed onto computer disk for analysis. Analysis of the data proceeded alongside the data collection or fieldwork. Ongoing analysis of the data would be supplemented by a further check of the transcripts after the completion of the fieldwork. Thirty-six midwives acted as informants in this project, of whom thirty-two had experienced the death of a mother in their care.

The midwife's experience of being supported, not being supported or occasionally providing support, emerged as major themes in this research project. The picture was, however, complicated by the multiplicity of different aspects of this phenomenon which the midwives raised. In spite of this and its variety of experiences, the group was quite homogeneous in its views regarding the benefits of support.

Collegial support

The most highly valued support which could be identified and utilised by the midwife following the death of a mother was that which was provided on an informal basis by her midwife colleagues. This finding is comparable with the observation of the benefits of 'mutual support' (Stapleton *et al.*, 1998: 142) and 'fellow workers' support' (Munro *et al.*, 1998) as mentioned earlier in this chapter. The form which this support assumes may have been little more than a brief 'How's things?' in passing in the corridor. Alternatively, it may have been in the form of a few tears shared in the quiet of the staff coffee room.

The collegial support did not necessarily need to be real. The potential for support or the perception of that support may have been sufficient. This often took the form of colleagues exchanging phone numbers with genuine encouragement to make contact if needed (Munro *et al.*, 1998; Metts *et al.*, 1994):

> 'And those of us who are kind of late 40s and have seen it before – we try really hard if there's a junior staff midwife involved to say "Look, here's my home phone number...".'
>
> (Midwife 13)

Occasionally for a minority of midwives this collegial support was not felt to be forthcoming. Such a lack of support applied to Midwife 12 who was so seriously affected by the experience that she became unwell and withdrew from midwifery practice for a while. It also applied to Midwife 28 who temporarily had been thought to be practising negligently: she felt unsupported to the point of ostracism for the few days while the standard of her practice was being seriously questioned:

> 'First of all there was no support for me, but when it was found that I was not to blame, all the people around were more supportive of me. The only support I had was the head nurse who was supportive throughout – right from the start and also my two close friends. The memory of it has stayed there ever since and it always will be with me.'

(Midwife 28)

For midwives such as Midwife 28, where collegial support was unforthcoming, the occupational and social isolation which the midwife inevitably seems to feel as a result of this rare event was seriously aggravated (Sarason *et al.*, 1994; Hingley & Marks,1991):

> 'But I found it quite an isolating situation. Because maternal death isn't something that happens every day, thank the Lord, and I found it isolating because people would come to me and say "I don't know what to say to you because this hasn't happened to me and I don't know how you're feeling" and a lot of people actually wrote that down.'

(Midwife 12)

A form of support which emerged as particularly valuable was that which arose out of the shared experience of those midwives who had actually been present when a mother died. Usually this shared experience related to one particular woman's death, but for some midwives it applied to events which may have been separated by years and continents:

> 'I think the midwife who was the senior midwife, she was very understanding. Probably because she'd been there for many years but she's retired now. She'd had a maternal death about five years previously and so she had experienced what I was going through.'
> RM: 'Her experience equated with yours?'
> 'Yes, Yes. And she spent a great deal of time with me.'

(Midwife 22)

The midwife who found the support of another who had had a similar experience appreciated the insights which they were able to share. This need to share the experience applied more particularly to those who may have cared for one mother around the time of her death. Thus, the sharing of the experience of loss emerged as very supportive to the midwife who was seeking to recover from the death of a mother:

'Just after her death I had a strong feeling of wanting to be more with the colleagues who were there at the time. . . . After the shift finished I found that I wanted to be with my colleagues who had shared that experience. There was a need for us to be together. We just sat there and did not do anything. There was some tea made, but it did not get poured. We did not want to leave. It was really a case of just being together. We were all very shocked and quiet. The affected staff were keeping close. Our feelings were such that could not be shared with others. The feelings were too raw to share. The affected group kept close together.'

(Midwife 4)

'I found it a lot easier to talk to midwives and to take their sympathy if they'd either been there on the day it happened and worked with me through that day or worked with [the woman] the two or three days before. I found it much more difficult to talk to people who did not even know [the woman] even though they were being really good and trying to be very supportive as well in the best way that they knew how.'

(Midwife 12)

This 'closed circle' of experienced midwives was clearly supportive to those who were part of it, but for some midwives being or not being involved in a particular incident became divisive. These divisions emerged in the form of criticism of those who were involved, as reported to me by a non-clinical midwife who had been closely involved with the death of a mother and who had sought to deal with these divisions in the staff of the maternity unit:

'. . . after it had happened some of the other midwives in the unit who weren't there on that Sunday, or the Monday, y'know were passing comments. "Oh well yes of course she was in pain or they should've done so and so" . . . or whatever or "Yes, well, I know [the family] and they are going to complain". And that was quite hurtful. I said "You weren't there at the time, you don't know what was happening and if you can't say anything constructive . . ."'

(Midwife 18)

The community midwife

There is an increased vulnerability when the midwife works partly or wholly in a community setting. Her vulnerability relates to the greater discrepancy between her need for support as compared with the fewer opportunities for her support needs to be met. This is partly because of her work being more solitary and also because she is less likely to be supported through informal passing encounters with knowledgeable and sympathetic colleagues. Her vulnerability is further increased when the news of the mother's death becomes public knowledge in the local community in which she lives and/or practises:

'When you're working in the community you're not surrounded by colleagues. I think that it must be easier when you happen across a colleague rather than having to make an appointment – the moment may have passed then.

'... My feelings, though, were anger and disbelief at what had happened. This was made worse by my having had personal contact with the family. I have been working as a community midwife and she was not my client. I knew the woman through my daughter, who goes to the same school as the woman's older daughter. There were things like the parent's association, where there was a lot of grief – so much so that I could not put my uniform on to take my daughter to school...'

RM: 'Was there any opportunity for you and your colleagues to share your feelings?'

'No we can't share our feelings because the staffing is so spread out and there's not much opportunity to see each other for these kinds of things.'

(Midwife 3)

'As well as all that, it turned out that the husband doesn't live very far from me – well he doesn't know where I live. He just lives a few streets away. So there is the community thing. People know that I'm a midwife – though I don't work in this area, thankfully. I've tried to keep myself out of it because people know ... My friend's sister's daughter is helping with the [baby]. So I try to keep out of it, because I know that the ward is having some difficulty with the family now. So I try to keep a fairly low profile from that point of view. I do not wish people to ask me anything about it. I do not know the details and I do not want to know – in case of questions. I don't want to get involved and people would be saying "She said 'Blah Blah Blah'".'

(Midwife 7)

Counselling

In view of the overwhelming importance which the midwives attached to collegial support, the role of the counsellor and counselling was less than clear. Many of the midwives considered that because counselling was neither widely nor easily available the midwife's recovery from the death of a mother was made more difficult. For the small number of midwives for whom professional counselling was available, it was generally considered inappropriate to take advantage of it. Midwives who decided not to accept counselling did so on the grounds that they preferred the support of colleagues who were knowledgeable about the circumstances of the particular event or, at least, the meaning of the death of a mother to a midwife:

'I don't know whether they [saw the counsellor]. None of the staff mentioned having been to her and they probably would have if they had. As far as I'm aware no one did contact her. This may have been our own fault. It might have been that she was not a midwife and might not have understood. She would not have that experience. She might not have been easy to talk to – not like talking to other midwives. It was as if midwives knew what it was all about – they were sharing their experience in every sense. It was such a shock and everybody talked about it. It was as if we did our own counselling – the counsellor was not needed.'

(Midwife 8)

'At the time that it happened I was very well supported from my colleagues and the consultants at work and everybody who was actually involved in the incident was very very supportive and really helped me a lot and was coming round to see me when I was off sick. Y'know being very very nice and at that time I didn't feel I could talk to an outsider about it. I wanted to talk to people who knew [the woman] like I knew her – the midwife who looked after her for the two to three days before I met her. And I wanted to be with people who knew the situation rather than with people who didn't know and I felt wouldn't understand.'

(Midwife 12)

For an even smaller number of midwives counselling was said to be available, but the circumstances of its availability were such that that it was not acceptable to the midwife. Examples of the unacceptability of counselling included the midwife being required to pay for it or being required to be referred through her line manager:

'I think it was after the lady cardiac arrested in theatre some of the staff midwives were quite upset. [The midwife managers] told us we could be referred to one of the staff counsellors who, y'know, ordinarily help patients with their problems, but we would have to go through one of them in order to be referred. Well, come on, either the system is there or it's not there. Either the backup is there or it's not. No one's going to go to your manager and say "I think I need counselling. Could you refer me?" It defeats the whole purpose. On paper it looks as if we have got counselling and the back-up. In reality we don't – it's back to your own support systems.'

(Midwife 13)

On the other hand those midwives working in a situation where a formal method of support is not available regarded it as necessary:

'[a meeting] was organised by my [bereavement counsellor] colleague and one of the managers, the head of midwifery who was actually on duty at the time. It was the head of midwifery who was mainly responsible for organising the staff support. All of the staff attended this debriefing meeting, the domestics, the cleaners, the auxiliaries, the midwives and one of the junior medical staff, but not the consultant. It was an incredible meeting. Everybody contributed, it began with the head of midwifery briefly outlining what had happened. Then everybody recounted their experience and what part they played and how they were feeling. There were no interruptions and all the people there were able to talk freely. At the end of the meeting the offer was made of further counselling with a trained counsellor for anyone who wanted it. I don't know whether anybody did.'

(Midwife 4)

The vulnerable midwife

The midwife informants also told me of how they perceived and attempted to meet other midwives' needs for support. This applied to less experienced colleagues as well as to those who were more vulnerable for other reasons. Examples given to me include a midwife grieving the death of her own mother, a midwife who had recently suffered post natal depression or a midwife whose domestic relationship was not very supportive:

'...my mother's death was the end of a very long and productive life and it was in the natural order of things. If I had her back and I had to write it for her I wouldn't have written it any differently. So I'm content with that. I'm comfortable with that. I shall be all right. But with a young woman having her first baby is something you don't come to terms with especially – even though she's not a relative.'

(Midwife 17)

'It's funny 'cos [my colleague] is more experienced than me timewise and she – her problem is that she's had post natal depression and she hasn't really got over it – about six years before and she wasn't right with that and she's still not right with that. There's been lots of other things happened apart from that. So I think that she's well-experienced but she's not done anything more. I've ... and I feel that I'm more confident in my practice and I've. . . . I've built myself up to a certain level so I know what I'm doing – I'm all right.'

(Midwife 10)

'I helped my colleague to sort out [the woman's] belongings and then I took [my colleague] home 'cos she lives by herself.'

(Midwife 18)

The unsupported midwife

The circumstances in which a midwife felt particularly unsupported were when her upset went unrecognised. An example is the community midwife who was required to continue to visit the new baby and the grieving family at home; another is when the midwife's caring relationship with the dying woman passed unnoticed by colleagues:

'The thing that bugged me mainly was that my care didn't seem to matter really, because the girl that had taken over in the afternoon had not known her like I did. But she was the one that was always associated with the death if you know what I mean. So it was sort of like – I was never part of it. It's like – I don't want to – I don't want recognition if you know what I mean. I don't want "You were the *one* that looked after her". The other girls they got "How're you doing?" sort of stuff and y'know I thought well how about me? (Laugh) But, like, she read the post mortem report, whereas I've never read it. Y'know it wasn't handed to me and it wasn't "How are you [midwife]?" '

(Midwife 25)

Organisational support

A number of organisational issues were raised by the midwives with whom I spoke. For many midwives the managerial support was plentiful and welcome, as one midwife told me:

'I must say that the managers [were] very good indeed. They arranged that a bereavement counsellor would be available to any of the staff who would like to contact her who had any involvement in her care regardless of whether it was minimal or major input. Also every midwife who was involved was sent a letter from the senior manager and we could go and talk to her or we could ring the counsellor. We really did have a lot of support at work. And the peer support was excellent, my colleagues were marvellous. A debriefing meeting was arranged to take place within 48 hours of when the lady died for the midwives and anyone else who wanted to go. That was very helpful.'

(Midwife 8)

For some midwives support is forthcoming from both managers and from supervisors of midwives. These managerial and supervisorial relationships may correspond to the examples of 'good practice' to which Stapleton and colleagues (1998) refer:

'Yes Yes. She spent a great deal of time with me.'
RM: 'Was she a manager?'
'She was a senior midwife of the old fashioned kind.'
RM: 'More like a middle manager?'
'Yeah.'
RM: 'Was she your supervisor as well as being your manager?'
'No. Although my supervisor was very supportive too.'

(Midwife 22)

While the midwives in clinical practice reported variable degrees of satisfaction with the support offered by their line managers, the non-clinical midwives' support was very different. The managers who spoke with me as 'experienced' midwives recounted their feelings of providing support for clinical practitioners in the absence of support from those in a line relationship above them. This lack of support from line managers and supervisors resonates with the problematical role model identified as being provided by many supervisors in Stapleton *et al.*'s (1998) study (see section 'Collegial support' earlier in this chapter):

'My boss was just coming back from holiday and it always seems as if something happens when she's away – it always does. And I sort of walked in – and I don't know whether it was the fact that she'd just got back from holiday or what but she said "Oh God! Now what's happened?" Y'know, but her whole attitude was "It's OK now that she's in ICU". Then she said "You can go home now and have a good sleep". I felt dreadful. It wasn't as if I'd been to an all night party. That's the last thing on my mind. She said, "Go! On you go now". I felt very let down at the time.'

(Midwife 18)

'As a manager, I had no one to call on. I had my supervisor, but because of [interpersonal things] I found myself in the situation of providing support for her. So my support was non-existent. I felt very isolated.'

(Midwife 2)

The experience of the manager in the event of maternal death is difficult to cope with but, as for any midwife, the supervisor may be expected to act as a resource. Unfortunately, as for any midwife, the manager may be disappointed. Additionally, the manager may be criticised by those to whom she is a manager and for whom she may also be expected to provide support. The manager's role in the mobilisation of support may be the focus of such adverse comments:

'There was some criticism from my colleagues that I was being ineffective – that I was not being supportive enough. I suppose that this was my colleagues being competitive since my promotion to a managerial post.

   It was very much a learning experience for all of us. I had to work out what was best for the future. I found out what was lacking and this was support. There was informal support. But a strong supportive framework was lacking. This reflects on midwifery supervision – there is a need for best practice guidelines. We all too often find that support is offered, but it is not given. There is a need for a side-by-side relationship between the midwife and the supervisor of midwives, which will provide support through emotional trauma, which is like an emotional eruption.'

(Midwife 2)

As has been observed not infrequently, because the midwife manager has often also been the supervisor of midwives the two roles may become blurred both in the mind of the supervisor as well as the midwife:

'Y'know, my supervisor when we have the annual interview she'll say "Why didn't you come and tell me this?" – whatever it was we were talking about? I just say, "I just wouldn't" – that's all. And she'd say, "But I'm your supervisor". I'd say, "Yes, but you're also my manager and I find the two positions in the one person quite incompatible". I've always said that every year as part of the annual supervisory interview. And I always say to her that I'm not happy that you're my manager plus my supervisor. I never know which hat she's wearing.'

(Midwife 13)

This confusion may be particularly hard for the clinical midwife who finds herself functioning temporarily as a manager as well as having to undertake her supervisorial duties. It may not be surprising that this midwife feels discontented that her need for support and her high level of functioning, in spite of this, pass unrecognised:

'I was working as the clinical midwife on the delivery suite, I was the manager for the whole unit and I was also the supervisor of midwives on call. I just thought "Oh gosh! What a responsibility!" And I think that made me feel that I had done a good job even though nobody said I had.

People – community midwives who came to the area to help us at the time – I wrote to everybody and thanked them all because I knew what a hard thing it was for everybody concerned. But personally I didn't feel that I got the appropriate amount of support from a more senior level. Not from my direct line manager anyway or from my supervisor of midwives. And that made it hard because I didn't feel that anybody ever said at any point "Thank you for everything that you did. You did a good job". Or anything like that. It was only when I wrote down my statement about it that I realised myself what an onerous task I'd had. And my support for one of the other midwives particularly who was directly involved has gone on.'

(Midwife 29)

The impression which remains is that some supervisors may not see this form of support as part of their supervisorial role. This perception may apply both to the support of the clinical midwife and to the support of the midwife-manager:

'The supervisors of midwives were not supportive [to me as a manager], though. They were not involved in the investigation. But I had the support of my opposite number, who was a non-midwife, for the debriefing.'

(Midwife 2)

'I was a very new midwifery manager and I learned very quickly about what was necessary. I had to make use of the existing supervisors. But because I had not been in post very long there were a lot of feelings about, which meant that they weren't very effective. The whole experience was devastating. I had expectations of the supervisors of midwives, that they would swing into action when this girl died, but they saw things differently.'

(Midwife 2)

This midwifery manager, in the same way as most of the experienced midwives who spoke to me, was able to glean certain important lessons from her experience of being involved with the death of a mother:

'Midwifery supervision, if it's going to work, needs to be strong and supportive and education oriented. The old style supervisors, who are still around, still tend to be discipline oriented.

But in this case supervision was lacking – the support for the midwives just did not happen. I suppose that the general situation must have made things more difficult. I mean that the fall-out due to it being my first managerial post – things did not go smoothly. The interpersonal things between me and the supervisors of midwives meant that the support for the midwives was spoiled and I had to do all the debriefing.'

(Midwife 2)

Other relevant issues arising out of the research

Time out

The extent to which peer support to avoid excessive stress and burnout manifests itself may be apparent in colleagues' offers of 'time out'. This has been discussed in the context of HIV care (earlier in this chapter) as 'mental health days' (Burr, 1996). Whether such basic human consideration is feasible in the maternity area in the event of the death of a mother became apparent in the study. For some midwives, such as one who was on night duty, time for recuperation was offered:

'The others took over our work on the ward – we didn't have many people in. Me and the other midwife – the two of us midwives just sat and cried. By the time we got sorted out it was five o'clock and we went off duty at seven. . . . We had . . . I came in later in the morning – I couldn't sleep. I spoke to the supervisor of midwives and the manager. We went over things and I wrote something down about what had happened. They were very nice, they let me have the next night off – I didn't even have to ask for it. They just said don't come in tonight. I only worked two nights a week.'

(Midwife 10)

'I couldn't work for the rest of that day that's for sure. 'Cos I couldn't cope with going back into another labouring woman at all, which we didn't have to because we'd already been kind of excused so to speak. 'Cos we'd had so much to do.'

(Midwife 27)

When I questioned midwives about the possibility of time out I was usually told that it was not wanted on the grounds that 'getting back to work' was a helpful coping strategy:

'. . . my confidence was shaken by this experience. It was so bad that I did not want to go back to work after this happened. I was due to have 2–3 nights off immediately after – and I did. When I came back I found that my colleagues were very considerate and protective towards me.'

(Midwife 20)

For other midwives, though, the culture of 'service and sacrifice' to which Kirkham (1999, 2000) refers (see section 'Culture' earlier in this chapter) seems to underpin this decision. As a supervisor of midwives explained to me:

> 'After all we did have a death before – one of the other supervisors was involved – another woman who had a stillbirth and then she bled and she died on the unit. And the supervisor said that she found that quite traumatic and she went off – she took three or four days off. She said, "I can't cope with this". And at the time I thought, "That is our job really to be there with the midwives. It's important that we're there to support the midwives". I was quite conscious of the need for me to be there for the staff and I think that I could do it for the staff.'
>
> (Midwife 18)

Funeral attendance

While potentially helpful for staff involved in a death (see section 'Nurses' support' earlier in this chapter), attending the funeral engenders certain misgivings and possibly difficulties (Burr, 1996; Mander, 1994). These difficulties became apparent in the context of the death of a mother, when the midwife was often discouraged from attending, both by the family and by midwifery managers:

> 'I know [the woman's father] recognises me. I know he knows me, but I just don't know what to say. It's like I wanted to go to the funeral. I talked to one of the [midwifery] sisters about it and she said that I should wait to be invited. They don't send invites to things like that though do they? . . . That was a very emotional part of their lives I s'pose really. That's why I wanted to go to the funeral as well. Or I wanted to write a card to just say – I never told them that I was sorry for them – not sorry for them, but – y'know how you do. But I was never allowed to do that because it would reflect badly on the unit. They would perhaps think we were admitting liability.'
>
> RM: 'Was this a management decision?'
>
> 'It was the sister who was on that day, she'd been on the previous night too. I didn't [go] because she'd said "No". I didn't push it. I took it at face value – that's what we do. You don't go interfering with people's grief. That's what the hospital says you have to do.'
>
> (Midwife 25)

Family and friends

The significant others of staff who are under stress have been reported in the literature (see section 'Nurses' support' earlier in this chapter) as being variably important in providing support (Burr, 1996; Etzion, 1984).

In my study, however, their contribution was consistently of less significance than that of colleagues. The presence of children though, as found by Sandall (1999), tended to act as a buffer against stress:

RM: 'Your small children – were they helpful?'

'Yes they were, they were actually staying with me Mum. They sleep at my mother's when I'm at work. And when I finished work I just wanted to see them. I just wanted to give them a cuddle. So I went to my Mum's and the kids could see I was upset and they were very nice. They didn't understand what was going on but I had a chat with me Mum and she was very good. She just let me gabble on. She doesn't understand the half of what you're saying but she lets you gabble on and get it out your system.'

(Midwife 10)

For one community midwife, her domestic support fulfilled the support need which arose out of the lack of convenient colleagues:

'I don't know how much support there has been on the ward. No one has spoken to me about it at all. I spoke with my family at home and that has helped. I felt that I'd got to talk to someone about it and when I read your article I thought that – this is it.'

RM: 'Your family...?'

'That's my husband. I don't need him to say anything, I just need him to listen to me. That's how I cope. He does not have to say anything. He does not need to comment, maybe he'll just say, "That's awful" or something like that. That's all I need. Some people say that their pets are like that – someone to talk to.'

(Midwife 7)

Summary

In summary, we should consider the extent to which the midwives who spoke with me were able to utilise the four strategies identified to maintain healthy relationships in a challenging clinical situation as mentioned in the earlier section 'Midwives and burnout' (Foster, 1996).

(1) *Promotion of team spirit* happened largely on an informal basis. This was when certain midwives responded spontaneously to the needs which they perceived among their colleagues and to which they were in a position to respond. The general view was that among midwife managers, such activities were not a priority, though there were exceptions to this observation.

(2) *Formal staff counselling training* also tended to be at the initiative of the individual midwife:

'I am currently doing a counselling course and was attending the course the following day. I feel that I was lucky that ... this helped me to process the experience.'   (Midwife 7)

(3) *Management support*, as indicated above is very variable and certain groups of midwives, such as those who work in management or in the community, are particularly vulnerable.

(4)   *Counselling for the counsellors (supervision)* is similarly dependent on the view that the individual supervisor takes of her role in this respect.

This less than ideal picture of the support available to midwives by midwives shows a distinct contrast to what is widely assumed to be available. Those experienced midwives whose experience of the death of a mother is distant in terms of time and/or place told me that they assumed that their experience would have been different, by which they meant less traumatic, had it occurred in the UK at the present time. That some of the UK experiences I was told about were very recent does not support this assumption. One midwife who had been retired for ten years when she wrote to me stated:

> 'Nowadays meetings are held for medical and midwifery staff and all matters appertaining to the maternal death are discussed.'
>
> (Midwife 15)

An experienced midwife whose experience was in another country was similarly certain:

> 'If it'd happened in this country and I'd been here I don't think, y'know, I wouldn't have just forgotten about it, but I don't think I would've felt like I do. . . .
> 'Like I mentioned before, I'm sure that if the incident had happened in this country the support I'd've had – it just wouldn't have happened – it wouldn't have been the same. I would have had a lot more support in this country. I would have got through it better.'
>
> (Midwife 28)

On the basis of this small research project, it is necessary to contemplate whether this impression of support in this particularly extreme situation may reflect a more general picture in everyday intraprofessional relationships. It may be appropriate to summarise the findings of this study as supporting the concept of 'emotional work'. This concept, introduced by Hochschild (1979), has been used in a range of nursing situations, but less in midwifery. It is based on the need for an individual to cope with others' painful feelings in the course of their job. In this way the employee is giving not just her standard 37.5 hours, but something of herself, which is essentially personal in addition to that for which she is contracted. It may be that this emotional labour of the midwife needs to be explicitly recognised in the form of reimbursement in kind; this involves ensuring good support for midwifery staff.

Chapter 8
Conclusion

I have attempted in this book to reflect on just one aspect of the way that care is provided for the childbearing woman at the beginning of the third millennium: the provision of social support, through a system of maternity care. The book began with a global picture of support and its benefits and challenges. I then moved on to focus more closely on the topic, first by examining the support provided by differing systems of health care. Next came support in the woman's complete experience of childbearing, then support by the midwife and, lastly, the provision of support in labour and childbirth. This gradually more precise focus led inexorably to an examination of the role of one particular person who has been recommended to provide care in childbirth. Though all too often neglected, I gave some attention in Chapter 7 to the needs of the staff who provide support for the childbearing woman, her family and, hopefully, each other.

In this concluding chapter I, first, summarise my analysis of the provision of support in childbearing. I then move on to consider the applicability of the relevant research and the recommendations emanating from it. On the basis of this background, certain comparisons seem germane and it is these, together with the context, which lead to my final conclusions.

Analysis of the situation

The introduction of this book provided me with an opportunity to adopt a heretical view of social support. I questioned whether its wide acceptance may be associated with it being a fashionable innovation which, like others in the past, have been welcomed as a universal remedy or panacea. In the first chapter I discussed the research in a range of settings which have suggested the effectiveness of support as a health care intervention. Social support has the additional benefit that it is relatively free of harmful side effects, which may be described as being 'iatrogenic'. In health care systems throughout the world, as discussed in Chapter 2, increasing costs are emerging as a major concern. Maternity care is in no way immune from this problem. These costs are associated, particularly in settings where the midwife is weak or non-existent, with an escalating medicalisation of childbearing. Scott and colleagues (1999) demonstrated that maternity care costs may not be amenable to the usual economies of scale, such as featured in the Botswana RCT (Madi *et al.*, 1999). This meta-analysis suggests that the practice of increasing the number of labouring women for whom each staff member cares is more than likely to be counterproductive in terms of financial costs:

'A high patient to nurse ratio may actually raise expenditures, rather than reducing costs, by increasing the need for unnecessary medical interventions'.

(Scott *et al.*, 1999: 1059)

A crucial aspect of the medicalisation of childbearing is the removal of the woman from her own environment. The birth then happens in an institutional setting which is dominated by professional carers who are largely strangers to the woman. It may be that more medical intervention has aggravated the increase in maternity health costs, which may accrue to individuals and/or the state and/or other agencies. In order to resolve this problem a low cost intervention has been sought by the medical fraternity. As well as being low cost, this solution is also required to be harmless to the extent that it will not compound the situation by engendering further iatrogenesis. The doula, whose characteristics and role have been scrutinised in Chapter 6, constitutes this low cost, low harm intervention. An added bonus is that her existence is thought to further lower costs, while exerting no threat to medical power. Thus, the doula presents no challenge to the status quo, and she offers no impediment to the further medicalisation of childbearing. It is becoming abundantly clear that the introduction and promotion of the doula may represent little more than a medically-inspired solution to the iatrogenic and other problems associated with the increasing medicalisation of childbearing.

The relevance of the research

The research, which underpins this analysis and the developments and recommendations outlined in this book, comprises a series of randomised controlled trials. The relevance, and thus the generalisability, of these RCTs needs to be called into question for two reasons. First, these studies were largely undertaken in third world settings. If not actually third world, the settings provided standards of care, as described by the researchers, which were low to the point of being sub-human. It may not be coincidental that these research settings featured health care systems in which the midwife did not exist, or where she had been driven out of existence or where she was prevented from practising to the full her unique skills. By this I mean those skills which feature the midwife offering social support by being 'with woman'.

Thus, the research findings may be less than relevant to those health care systems where the midwife has survived, with at least the potential to practise, or may even have flourished (see section on 'The Netherlands' in Chapter 2). The research is further limited in its applicability by the precise settings in which it was undertaken. This relates to the institutions, which were invariably hospitals, and the systems of care, which were invariably and powerfully medically dominated.

In contrast to this well documented picture of institutionalised childbirth, there is a notable lack of research evidence relating to the support needs of the woman giving birth in her own home. This deficit may possibly be associated with the limited number of women who are in a position to choose to give birth at home. Alternatively, the deficit may be due to the redundancy of such research because, as has been identified in an evidence-based publication:

> 'At home it is common practice for midwives to provide continuous care.'
>
> (MIDIRS, 1996: 6)

Although information about the benefits of support in labour is plentiful, the lack of research into the provision of support at home is just one example of areas which are still in need of research. Thus the research evidence is in no way complete. A further example of an area of need is found in the evidence base, which varies hugely in the level of instruction given to the support person. This variation extends from the advice to use her 'personal resources' (Hofmeyr & Nikodem, 1996: 92) to the person being a fully qualified nurse and midwife, as in the Dublin regime (O'Driscoll *et al.*, 1993). It is hardly surprising, therefore, that more research is recommended in order to find out what the support person actually does or does not do to ensure that her support is effective (MIDIRS, 1996: 6). Additionally, the same publication recommends that the personal characteristics need to be elucidated, as outlined in Chapter 6.

The research which has been published has focused largely on the organisational aspects and the pathophysiological effects of the provision of support. The findings have been assessed in terms of the easily measurable outcomes, such as those which may be counted. Little attention has been given to the experience of the woman who is in a position to enjoy the benefits of being supported. As mentioned in the section 'The significance of the doula' in Chapter 6, if the care of the woman in labour is to be genuinely woman-centred, it is vital that the woman, probably through women's consumer groups, is involved in policy decision-making. In this way it is more likely that her views are sought, that her voice is heard and that a suitable policy response is made.

Comparable scenarios

The picture which has been presented here has resulted in the recommendation for a change to be introduced to a system of care (Hodnett, 2000c). A systems approach to examine any phenomenon involves its total relationships, rather just studying it in isolation. Thus, it is recognised that by altering one aspect of that phenomenon which is a system, it is inevitable that other aspects will also be changed (Buckley, 1968). In a number of situations relating to maternity care certain changes which have been planned and introduced with the expectation of particular benefits, have ultimately proved to have other rather different outcomes. It may be helpful to contemplate these comparable scenarios in order to evaluate the significance of the current recommendations.

Historical scenarios

Whereas some of the less than beneficial outcomes are ongoing, others have occurred in the more distant or more recent past.

The Midwives Act 1902

One of these situations was mentioned in Chapter 2: the passage of the Ninth Midwives Bill to become the Midwives Act of 1902 in England. This much sought after legislation was originally intended to benefit the childbearing woman by protecting the public from midwifery practice which fell short of the then currently accepted standards. It was also hoped to enhance the status of the midwife by encouraging her to be recognised as a respected professional. Whether the first aim was achieved is not easy to judge because it is not known how many bona fide and uncertificated midwives continued to practise long after the enactment (Towler & Bramall, 1986). It is, however, well established that the second aim was not achieved. This was due partly to the ongoing hostility among medical practitioners at grass roots level and partly to the overpowering medical majority on the Central Midwives Boards (Donnison, 1988). Thus, this legislation had the reverse effect from that which was intended, by delivering the control of the midwifery profession into the hands of the midwife's major competitors.

The UK National Health Service and hospital birth

Another example of an unexpected outcome from a development which the midwife anticipated as being totally beneficial for the woman in her care was the introduction of the UK National Health Service (NHS) in 1948 (Tew, 1995). The midwife, like the woman, welcomed the free maternity care in hospital offered through the NHS. It was foreseen as an opportunity for the woman to be given safe care in a restful environment, away from the nagging demands of family and domestic drudgery. Tew recounts how medical practitioners welcomed the advent of the NHS for very different reasons. To the obstetrician the NHS maternity hospital allowed him to test out the 'developing theories about the advantages of their style of management [of labour]' (Tew, 1995: 71). The transfer of uncomplicated childbearing from the home to the hospital, which was hastened by the introduction of the NHS, undermined the midwife's traditional power-base to the point of 'extinction' (Webster, 2000). Once more, that power was delivered directly into the hands of the midwife's major competitors.

Active management of labour

One of the consequences of the increased hospitalisation of childbirth started to become apparent in the early 1970s. This is the medical practitioner's greater use of, first, interventions to induce labour and, second, active management to speed up labour which has begun spontaneously. Subsequently these latter practices became known as acceleration or augmentation of labour (O'Driscoll *et al.*, 1973). The use of artificial rupture of the membranes and oxytocic drugs to achieve these ends was initially welcomed by the midwife. My memory tells me that the midwife at that time was well aware of the hazards of prolonged labour for the woman and the baby. The midwife allowed herself to be persuaded that shortening pregnancy, the first stage, the second stage and the third stage of labour could, logically, avoid prolonged labour. This logical outcome could, she believed, only benefit the woman and baby. In line with the Dublin regime, no evidence was produced to substantiate these claims. By the time that evidence started to become available these interventions had achieved the status of standard practice and were often included in what was termed 'normal' childbirth. Unfortunately, by that time it was too late to put the genie back into the bottle and the midwife's role had been reduced to little more than that of an obstetric nurse (Walker, 1976).

Episiotomy

While not usually included as a method of active management, a further intervention frequently employed by the midwife also serves as an example of an intended benefit to the childbearing woman. The surgical incision of the perineum to facilitate the birth, usually known as episiotomy, was forbidden to the midwife until 1967 (Robinson *et al.*, 1983). The lifting of this veto, the increasing hospitalisation of birth and the commitment to active management of labour among medical practitioners were some of the factors which increased the likelihood of this form of surgery (Graham, 1997: 78). According to Graham's study of episiotomy as an example of obstetric intervention, a more insidious and possibly more important factor was the midwife's deference to medical authority. Yet again, the midwife allowed herself to be persuaded by the logic of an unsubstantiated medical argument. The integrity of the woman's pelvic floor, she was told, could be preserved in this way. Additionally, the 'ignominy' of a third degree or complete perineal tear could be avoided (Graham, 1997: 76). That the fundamental midwifery skill of 'guarding the perineum' was being sabotaged passed largely unmentioned. In spite of a few dissenting voices, this intervention was widely used on a routine basis. Fortunately the randomised controlled trial undertaken by Sleep (1984) provided the evidence to reverse this pattern. Her RCT demonstrated that there was certainly no clear fetal or maternal benefit in the widespread practice of episiotomy. Thus, the episiotomy saga shows how the practice of the midwife was once again manipulated by her medical colleagues. The outcome of this sorry saga featured no benefits for the childbearing woman or her baby (Sleep, 1984). The price paid by the midwife, however, was a further reduction in her professional autonomy.

Ongoing scenarios

So far historical scenarios have been presented to demonstrate how change may have harmful effects which are at odds with the anticipated benefits. Other examples are ongoing or forthcoming.

The lactation consultant

An innovative role which merits attention is a transatlantic import which has so far attracted limited attention in the media devoted to childbearing. This person has styled herself the 'lactation consultant', although that seems to be one of the few features of this person on which her advocates appear to agree. In the UK midwifery media the lactation consultant has been introduced as some kind of superwoman by Cullen (1999). This person is clearly very different from a clinical midwifery practitioner. The author identifies her role as being to act as a change agent. She has a responsibility for the education of both midwifery students and midwifery practitioners.

The UK picture presented by Finigan (1996), on the other hand, describes in more realistic terms a midwife who is also qualified as a lactation consultant. This clinical midwife describes how the weaknesses of her midwifery education required her to undertake this course of action in order to practise the fundamental midwifery skill of assisting a new mother to initiate breast feeding. She reports how it is all too often necessary for the midwife to draw on her own personal experience of breast feeding if she is to be able to help the new mother at all. According to Finigan her education on breast feeding comprised only anatomy and physiology, without any attention to the processes, the principles, the research or the counselling skills. That so little attention is given to this crucial midwifery skill during midwifery education is a sad reflection on that educational system. This sorry picture may resonate with the undervaluing of the midwifery care of the perineum known as 'guarding' in the episiotomy saga mentioned above.

A USA publication by Lauwers and Shinskie (2000) presents a picture of the lactation consultant which is different again. This practitioner's role is reflected in the authors' use of the word 'counseling' to indicate the care which she provides. This includes care in the broadest sense of the word, verging on holism, with a definite emphasis on the teaching and support of the breast feeding woman. This good news also has another side to it which may be disconcerting. This aspect appears with the authors' introduction of the 'lactation consulting profession', and the International Lactation Consultant Association. Thus, it becomes apparent that the professionalisation of this group of practitioners is well-advanced. It may be that the lactation consultant is necessary in the North American health care system because, as has been explained elsewhere, breast feeding 'falls between the cracks between pediatric and obstetrical care' (Riordan & Auerbach, 2000: 1). Thus, because there the person with the responsibility for providing support for this woman at this time has been driven out of existence and because the traditional family and social supports no longer operate, it has been necessary to invent a practitioner to fulfil this function.

The advent of the lactation consultant raises a number of issues. The first relates to the system of health care in which she practises. It is clear that she may be needed in settings where 'cracks' divide the services which are provided for the childbearing woman. Other health care systems, though, are different and may not face these difficulties. Thus her relevance to the UK situation may need to be questioned.

A second issue raised by the advocacy of Lauwers and Shinskie for the lactation consultant relates, in more general terms, to the North American enthusiasm to export aspects of their culture. The lay media may be one example where a superficially common language has served to facilitate the export of an assumption of a common culture across the Atlantic. It may be that the unidirectional nature of this flow results in perceptions which give rise to words like 'protectionism'. A significant example of this export relates to the health care culture. Welcomed by some was the application of Enthoven's (1994) market economics to the UK health care system. This resulted in many of the NHS reforms introduced by the Conservative Government of 1979–97. The unidirectional nature of the movement of knowledge is clearly apparent in the area of childbearing knowledge (Garcia, 1993). A similar phenomenon has been identified in nursing education through academic nursing publications (McConnell, 2000). In this context, too, it may be helpful to contemplate whether this transfer of material is welcome and whether the welcome also extends to the ideas and values which the material transmits.

Having questioned whether the lactation consultant has a place in the UK health care system, it is necessary to examine the conditions under which the import of this expert would be a possibility. There is no doubt that the midwife is well able to provide the support which the breast feeding woman needs if she is to successfully initiate and establish her lactation. It may be that the only phenomenon which prevents the midwife from providing this support is the demands of the organisation of the health care system within which she functions. In the post natal ward increasing numbers of women recovering from a surgical birth urgently require a high standard of nursing care. It is unfortunate that due to limited resources these requirements may supersede the support needs of the healthy woman initiating a physiological function such as breast feeding. The general move towards community care is widely associated with encouraging the woman to accept early discharge from the busy maternity unit into the care of the equally busy community midwife. Thus, although lip service may be paid to increasing breast feeding rates and duration, managerial priorities may be preventing the midwife from spending the time needed with the new mother in either setting. In this way it becomes apparent that another care provider is likely to be necessary. The lactation consultant is waiting in the wings ready to step into this gap in the service provision.

The doula

In the same way that the lactation consultant may be awaiting her moment to move centre stage, the doula is also ready to play her part in the clearly beneficial provision of support in labour. Her advent is based on the authoritative labour support research literature featuring a one-to-one relationship, which is the traditional role of the midwife. The midwife, however, is increasingly being prevented from offering such personalised support for the very reason that it is ever more necessary – the more extreme and more pervasive medicalisation of childbearing.

It may be, therefore, that the midwife finds herself in what has been referred to as a 'double whammy'. The midwife is being required, by the research evidence, to achieve certain high standards of care. At the same time, however, the necessary resources which would enable her to provide that care are being withdrawn from the midwife practising within the UK health care system. The likelihood is that, by way of a solution to this apparently intractable problem, a new invention in the form of the doula is to be parachuted in. The doula carries the benefits of being relatively cheap, non-threatening to the medical power-base and 'scientifically-proven'. Unfortunately, unlike the doula, the midwife and the care which she provides have not been subjected to randomised controlled trials. There may even be uncertainty about what the midwife actually does. Unlike the nurse in the North American labour and delivery area, the UK midwife has not been subjected to the type of work-sampling studies which were undertaken in Canada (Gagnon & Waghorn, 1996). Thus, the midwife has not established her effectiveness in a way which meets the requirements of the current evidence-based dogma. It may not even be possible to state unequivocally that the midwife and her practice have stood the test of time. The midwife tends to assume that the care which she provides constitutes support, but the evidence for this assumption may be called into question. In fact the reverse may be true, in that some fundamental aspects of midwifery care may not be recognised as valuable by the midwife who provides that care.

While it may seem that the doula constitutes a threat to the midwife and to midwifery practice, this may not necessarily be the case. The doula is not the problem. In fact, the doula is little more than a symptom or a remedy for the situation which has arisen. The underlying problem relates, not to the doula, but to the reasons for which she is being accepted, welcomed and promoted. The doula is being used or even manipulated by her inventors and advocates, who are the medical practitioners. The reasons for her invention relate to the twin problems of medical intervention and the associated costs, the latter of which includes both financial costs and health costs.

Conclusion

I have been advancing the argument that the role and the existence of the midwife may be under threat. This threat may not necessarily be in the form of a new arrival in the birthing room. It is more likely that the threat is from the midwife's long term adversary, in that the medical practitioner is proposing a cheaper, less authoritative, less threatening and scientifically endorsed 'changeling' to supplant the midwife.

In the earlier sections of this chapter, I have suggested that one of the strengths of the midwife is that she is good at providing care with little thought for her own welfare. Thus, the midwife may not be most astute at recognising those phenomena which will eventually adversely affect her role and functioning. My examples of midwifery legislation, the introduction of the NHS, hospital birth, active management of labour and episiotomy suggest that the midwife only realises the implications of innovation for her occupational role when it is too late.

The doula and her advocates may effectively be pushing at an open door because the midwife is not making full use of the opportunities which are available to her, as has been demonstrated by research into the care that she provides during labour. The study by Spiby and colleagues (1999) shows the woman's high expectations that the midwife will provide effective support in labour. These researchers, however, illustrate the limited extent to which the midwife is prepared to meet these expectations. This shortfall is compensated for by the woman's partner assuming a surprisingly high profile. Similarly, the study in Aberdeen by Rennie and colleagues (1998) indicates the deteriorating importance of the midwife to the woman in association with the experience of birth. As found by Spiby and colleagues, the Aberdeen study also found that the woman's partner becomes reciprocally more significant. Thus the opportunities presented to the midwife to make a difference to the woman's birth experience fail to be fully utilised.

These midwife researchers' conclusions resonate with those of Odent. These were rehearsed in Chapter 6, and suggest that unless the midwife grasps and utilises the opportunities which present themselves to her, those opportunities will disappear. This may really be a case of 'use it or lose it'. As with the examples of change to which I have referred, such as active management and hospitalisation, the midwife should not wait until it is too late before asserting her unique ability to provide care at this crucial point in the life of the woman and her family. If the midwife and midwifery are to survive in the form in which they exist in the UK and New Zealand, it is necessary for the midwife to undertake research to establish that she performs a unique function and does so more effectively than any other occupational group. The benefits of the increasing knowledge about support in childbearing are obvious. The time is long overdue for looking closely at where this knowledge is leading.

References

Abbott, A. (1988) *The System of Professions*. Chicago, University of Chicago Press.

AIMS/NCT (1997) *A Charter for Ethical Research in Maternity Care*. London, AIMs/NCT.

Alexander, J. (1998) Confusing debriefing and defusing postnatally: the need for clarity of terms, purpose and value. *Midwifery*, **14**(2) 122–4.

Anderson, T. (2000) Maternal attitudes to amniotomy and labor duration: a critique. *MIDIRS Midwifery Digest*, **10**(2) 195–7.

Annie, C.L. & Groer, M. (1991) Childbirth stress: an immunologic study. *Journal of Obstetric Gynecologic & Neonatal Nursing*, **20**(5) 391–7.

Antonovsky, A. (1979) *Health Stress and Coping*. San Francisco, Jossey Bass.

Antonucci, T.C. (1985) Social Support: Theoretical advances, recent findings and pressing issues. In *Social Support Theory Research and Application* (eds I.G. Sarason & B.R. Sarason) pp. 21–37. Boston, Nijhoff.

Appleby, L., Warner, R., Whitton, A. & Faragher, B. (1997) A controlled study of fluoxetine and cognitive-behavioural counselling in the treatment of postnatal depression. *British Medical Journal*, **29** 314(7085) 932–6.

Arvidsson, G. (1995) Regulation of planned markets in health care. Chapter 3 in *Implementing Planned Markets in Health Care: Balancing Social and Economic Responsibility* (eds R.B. Saltman & C. Van Otter). Buckingham, Open University Press.

Audit Commission (1997) *First Class Delivery: Improving Maternity Services in England and Wales*. London, Audit Commission.

Baker, E., Israel, B. & Schurman, S. (1996) Role of control and support in occupational stress: an integrated model. *Social Science and Medicine*, **43**(7) 1145–59.

Bakker, R.H.C., Groenewegen, P.P., Jabaaij, L., Meijer, W., Sixma, H. & de Veer, A. (1996) 'Burnout' among Dutch midwives. *Midwifery*, **12**(4) 174–81.

Barber, T. (1998) Stress and the management of change. *RCM Midwives Journal*, **1**(1) 26–7.

Barrera, M. (1981) Social support in the adjustment of pregnant adolescents: assessment issues. In *Social Networks and Social Support* (ed. B.H. Gottlieb), vol 4 Sage Studies in Community Mental Health. Beverly Hills, Sage Publications.

Beail, N. & McGuire, J. (1982) *Fathers: Psychological Perspectives*. London, Junction Books.

Beake, S., McCourt, C., Page, L. & Vail, A. (1998) The use of clinical audit in evaluating maternity services reform: a clinical reflection. *Journal of Evaluation in Clinical Practice*, **4**(1) 75–83.

Beaton, J. & Gupton, A. (1990) Childbirth expectations: a qualitative analysis. *Midwifery*, **6**(3) 133–9.

Beaton, R.D., Murphy, S.A., Pike, K.C. & Corneil, W. (1997) Social support and network conflict in firefighters and paramedics. *Western Journal of Nursing Research*, **19**(3) 297–313.

Beaver, R.C., Sharp, E.S. & Cotsonis, G.A. (1986) Burnout experienced by nurse-midwives. *Journal of Nurse-Midwifery*, **31**(1) 13–15.

Bedford, V.A. & Johnson, N. (1988) The role of the father. *Midwifery*, **4**(4) 190–5.

Beech, B.L. (1993) Midwife supervision or victimisation? *Modern Midwife*, **3**(6) 44.

Benner, P. (1984) *From Novice to Expert: Excellence and Power in Clinical Nursing Practice.* Menlo Park, CA, Addison-Wesley.

Berkman, L.F. & Syme, S.L. (1979) Social networks, host resistance and mortality: a nine year follow up of Alameda county residents. *American Journal of Epidemiology*, **109**, 186–204.

Berry, L.M. (1988) Realistic expectations, of the labor coach. *Journal of Obstetric Gynecologic and Neonatal Nursing*, **17**(5) 354–5.

Bewley, C. (1997) Domestic violence and pregnancy. *Changing Childbirth Update*, **10**, 5.

Birch, E.R. (1986) The experience of touch received during labour. *Journal of Nurse-Midwifery*, **31**(6) 270–5.

Blazer, D. (1982) Social support and mortality in an elderly community population. *American Journal of Epidemiology*, **115**, 684–94.

Bourgeault, I.L. & Fynes, M. (1997) Integrating lay and nurse-midwifery into the US and Canadian health care systems. *Social Science & Medicine*, **44**(7) 1051–63.

Bower, H. (1993) Team midwifery in Oxford. *MIDIRS Midwifery Digest*, **3**(2) 143–5.

Brandom, E. (1996) Audit and research—basic principles. *Midwives*, **109**(1304) 255.

Briggs, A. (1972) *Report of the Committee on Nursing.* London, HMSO.

Bryanton, J., Fraser-Davey, H. & Sullivan, P. (1994) Women's perceptions of nursing support in labour. *Journal of Obstetric Gynecologic & Neonatal Nursing*, **23**(8) 638–44.

Buckley, W. (1968) *Modern Systems Research for the Behavioral Scientist.* Chicago, Aldine.

Bulger, R.J. (1999) Healing persons and therapeutic institutions. *American Journal of Obstetrics and Gynaecology*, **180**(4) 875–82.

Burnard, P. (1991) *Coping with Stress in the Health Professions: a practical guide.* London, Chapman & Hall.

Burr, C.K. (1996) Supporting the helpers. *Nursing Clinics of North America*, **31**(1) 243–51.

Burtch, B. (1994) *Trials of Labour: the re-emergence of midwifery.* Montreal, McGill-Queens University Press.

Butterworth, T. & Faugier, J. (1992) Supervision for life. In *Clinical Supervision and Mentorship in Nursing* (eds T. Butterworth & J. Faugier). London, Chapman & Hall.

Callaghan, P. & Morrissey, J. (1993) Social support and health: a review. *Journal of Advanced Nursing*, **18**(2) 203–10.

Campbell, R. (1997) Evaluating maternity care. Chapter 1, pp 1–13 in *The Organization of Maternity Care* (eds R. Campbell & J. Garcia). Hale, Hochland & Hochland.

Campero, L., Garcia, C., Diaz, C., Ortiz, O., Reynoso, S. & Langer, A. (1998) 'Alone, I wouldn't have known what to do' – a qualitative study on social support during labor and delivery in Mexico. *Social Science & Medicine*, **47**(3) 395–403.

Carr-Saunders, A.M. & Wilson, P.A. (1933) *The Professions.* Oxford, Clarendon Press.

Cassidy, P. (1999) The first stage of labour: physiology and early care. Chapter 21 in *Mylers Textbook for Midwives* (eds V.R. Bennett & L.K. Brown). Edinburgh, Churchill Livingstone.

Chambers, H.M. & Chan, F.Y. (2000) Support for women/families after perinatal death. *The Cochrane Database of Systematic Reviews* (issue 1). Cochrane Pregnancy and Childbirth Group, The Cochrane Library, The Cochrane Collaboration.

Changing Childbirth (1993) Part 1 Report of the Expert Maternity Group. London, The Stationery Office.

Cherniss, C. (1980) *Staff Burn-out: Job Stress in the Human Services.* London, Sage Publications.

Cheung, N.F. (1997) Chinese zuo yuezi (sitting in for the first month of the postnatal period) in Scotland. *Midwifery*, **13**(2) 55–65.

Clarke, J.B. (1999) Evidence-based practice: a retrograde step? The importance of pluralism in evidence generation for the practice of health care. *Journal of Clinical Nursing*, **8**(1) 89–94.

Coates, M–M. (1999) Tides in breastfeeding practice. Chapter 1, p. 3 in *Breastfeeding and Human Lactation* (eds J. Riordan & K.G. Auerbach) 2nd edn. Massachusetts, Jones & Bartlett.

Cobb, S. (1976) Social support as a moderator of life stress. *Psychosomatic Medicine*, **38**(5) 300–14.

Cochrane, A.L. (1972) *Effectiveness and Efficiency*. London, Nuffield Provincial Hospitals Trust.

Cohen, S. & Syme, S.L. (1985) *Social Support and Health*. Orlando, Academic Press.

Copstick, S., Hayes, R.W., Taylor, K.E. & Morris, N.F. (1985) A test of a common assumption regarding the use of antenatal training during labour. *Journal of Psychosomatic Research*, **20**, 215–18.

Corbett, C.A. & Callister, L.C. (2000) Nursing support during labour. *Clinical Nursing Research*, **9**(1) 70–83.

Coyne, J.C. & Delongis, A. (1986) Going beyond social support: The role of social relationships in adaptation. *Journal of Consulting and Clinical Psychology*, **54**, 454–60.

Crompton, J. (1996) Post traumatic stress disorder and childbirth. *British Journal of Midwifery*, **4**(6) 290–4.

Cullen, L. (1999) Lactation consultancy: enhancing midwifery practice? *RCM Midwives Journal*, **2**(3) 83.

Currell, R. (1996) The organisation of maternity care. In *Midwifery Practice Core Topics 1* (eds J. Alexander; V. Levy & S. Roch). London, Macmillan.

Curtis, J.M. (1995) Elements of critical incident debriefing. *Psychological Reports*, **77**(1) 91–6.

Cutrona, G.E. & Russell, D.W. (1990) Type of social support and specific stress: toward a theory of optimal matching. *Social Support and Interactional View* (eds. I.G. Sarason, B.R. Sarason & G.R. Pierce) pp. 319–66. New York, John Wiley & Sons.

Davies, J. (1990) Against the odds. *Nursing Times*, **86**(44) 29–31.

Davies, J. (1997a) The Newcastle community midwifery care project: The evaluation of the project. Chapter 4, pp. 115–140 in *Midwives Research and Childbirth*, (eds A.M. Thomson & S. Robinson) Vol. 2. London, Chapman & Hall.

Davies, J. (1997b) Them and us: poverty deprivation and maternity care. Chapter 4, p. 50–62, in *Challenges In Midwifery Care*, (eds I. Kargar & S.C. Hunt). Basingstoke, Macmillan.

Declercq, E. (1998) 'Changing Childbirth' in the United Kingdom: lessons for US health policy. *Journal Health Policy Politics & Law*, **23**(5) 833–59.

Declercq, E.R. (1994) A cross-national analysis of midwifery politics: six lessons for midwives. *Midwifery*, **10**(4) 232–7.

Deery, R. & Corby, D. (1996) A case for clinical supervision in midwifery. Chapter 14, p. 203, in *Supervision of Midwives* (ed. M. Kirkham). Hale, Books for Midwives Press.

Dekker, W. (1987) *Bereidheid tot Verandering*. Commissie Structur en Financiering Gezondheidszorg, Den Haag DOP.

Demilew, J. (1996) Independent midwives' views of supervision. Chapter 13, pp. 183–204, in *Supervision of Midwives* (ed. M. Kirkham). Hale, Books for Midwives Press.

DeVries, R. (1996) The midwife's place: an international comparison of the status of midwives. Chapter 13, pp. 159–74, in *Midwives and Safer Motherhood* (ed. S.F. Murray). London, Mosby.

DeVries, R.G. & Barroso, R. (1997) Midwives among the machines: re-creating midwifery in the late twentieth century. Chapter 12 in *Midwives Society and Childbirth: debates and controversies in the modern period* (eds H. Marland & A.M. Rafferty). London, Routledge.

DHSS (1976) *Sharing Resources*—Report of the Resource Allocation Working Party. London, The Stationery Office.

DHSS (1983) *The NHS Management Enquiry*. London, The Stationery Office.

Dickson, S.A. (1954) *Panacea, or, Precious Bane: Tobacco in Sixteenth Century Literature*. New York, New York Public Library,

DoH (1989) *Working for Patients: education and training*. London, Department of Health.

DoH (1993) *Changing Childbirth*: Report of the Expert Maternity Group. London, Department of Health.

DONA (1999) Doulas of North America Position Paper: *The Doula's contribution to modern maternity care*. Doulas of North America
http://www.dona.com/positionpapers.html

Donnison, J. (1988) *Midwives and Medical Men*, 2nd edn. London, Heinemann.

Downe, S. (1998) Birthwrite: Motherless mothers and social support. *British Journal of Midwifery*, **6**(10) 682.

Draper, J. (1997) Whose welfare in the labour room? A discussion of the increasing trend of fathers' birth attendance. *Midwifery*, **13**(3) 132–8.

Draper, J. (1998) Personal communication cited in (J. Sullivan-Lyons), Men becoming fathers: 'Sometimes I wonder how I'll cope'. Chapter 12 in *Psychological Perspectives on Pregnancy and Childbirth* (ed. S. Clement). Edinburgh, Churchill Livingstone.

Duck, S. & Perlman, D. (eds) (1985) *Understanding Personal Relationships: an inter-disciplinary approach*. London, Sage Publications.

Durkheim, E. (1951) *Suicide: a study in sociology*, (trans. J. A. Spalding & G. Simpson). Illinois, Glencoe Press.

Dyregrov, A. (1989) Caring for helpers in disaster situations: psychological debriefing. *Disaster Management*, **2**, 25–30.

Edelwich, J. & Brodsky, A. (1980) *Burn-Out*. New York, Human Sciences.

Edwards, N. (1996) Is everything rosy in the MSLC Garden? *AIMS Journal*, **8**(3) 6–9.

EEC (1980) *Midwives Directives*. Official Journal of the European Communities No. L133 of 11.2.80. London, The Stationery Office.

Elbourne, D., Oakley, A. & Chalmers, I. (1989) Social and psychological support during pregnancy, Chapter 15 in *Effective Care In Pregnancy And Childbirth* (eds. I. Chalmers, M. Enkin & M.J.N.C. Keirse) vol. 1. Oxford University Press.

Elliott, S.A. (1989) Psychological strategies in the prevention and treatment of postnatal depression. *Bailliere's Clinical Obstetrics and Gynaecology*, **3**(4) 879–903.

Enthoven, A.C. (1989) *Management information and analysis for the Swedish Health Care System*. Lund, The Swedish Institute for Health Economics.

Enthoven, A.C. (1994) On the ideal market structure for third party purchasing of health care. *Social Science & Medicine*, **39**(10) 1413–24.

Etzion, D. (1984) Moderating effect of social support on the stress-burnout relationship. *Journal of Applied Psychology*, **69**(4) 615–22.

Evans, F. (1997) The Newcastle community midwifery care project: The project in action. Chapter 4, pp. 104–114 in *Midwives Research and Childbirth*. (eds A.M. Thomson & S. Robinson) vol. 2. London, Chapman & Hall.

Fawcett, J., Tulman, L. & Myers, S. (1988) Development of the inventory of functional status after childbirth. *Journal of Nurse-Midwifery*, **33**(6) 252–60.

Fernandez, C.O., Canterino, J.C., Dambeck, S. & McKeever, J. (1999) *Cesarean delivery rate reduction*. 19th annual meeting of the Society for Maternal Fetal Medicine, San Francisco.

Finigan, V. (1996) ENB framework enhances midwifery practice. *Nursing Times*, **92**(33) 42–43 (MIDIRS **7**(1) 28–9).

Flamm, B.L. (2000) Cesarean section: A worldwide epidemic? *Birth*, **27**(2) 139–40.

Flamm, B.L., Berwick, D.M. & Kabcenell, A. (1998) Reducing cesarean section rates safely: lessons. *British Medical Journal*, **28**(298)(6668) 223–6.

Flint, C., Poulengeris, P. & Grant, A. (1989) The 'Know Your Midwife' scheme – a randomised trial of continuity of care by a team of midwives. *Midwifery*, **5**(1) 11–16.

Ford, G. Ecob, R., Hunt, K., Macintyre, S. & West, P. (1994) Patterns of class inequality in health through the lifespan. *Social Science & Medicine*, **39**(8) 1037–50.

Forrest, G.C., Standish, E. & Baum, J.D. (1982) Support after perinatal death: a study of support and counselling after perinatal bereavement. *British Medical Journal*, **285**(20) 1475–9.

Foster, A. (1996) Perinatal bereavement: Support for families and midwives. *Midwives*, **109**(1303) 218–9.

Francome, C., Savage, W., Churchill, H. & Lewison, H. (1993) *Caesarean Birth in Britain:*

A book for health professionals and parents. London, NCT, and Middlesex University Press.

Freidson, E. (1970) *Profession of Medicine.* New York, Mead & Co.

Friere, P. (1972) *The Pedagogy of the Oppressed.* Harmondsworth, Penguin.

Gagnon, A.J., Waghorn, K. & Covell, C. (1997) A randomized trial of one-to-one support of women in labor. *Birth*, June, **24**(2) 71–7.

Gagnon, A.J. & Waghorn, K. (1996) Supportive care by maternity nurses: a work sampling study in an intrapartum unit. *Birth*, **23**(1) 1–6.

Galbraith, S. (1998) A framework for clinical governance. June, Scottish Office Home & Health Departments. http://www.show.scot.nhs/gov/uk

Gamble, D. & Morse, J.M. (1993) Fathers of breastfed infants: postponing and types of involvement. *Journal of Obstetric Gynecologic and Neonatal Nursing*, **22**, 358 65.

Garcia, J. (1993) Encyclopedia of childbearing. *Birth*, **20**, 4225–6.

Garcia, J. (1999) Mothers' views and experiences of care. Chapter 6, p. 81 in *Community-based Maternity Care* (eds G. Marsh & M. Renfrew). Oxford, Oxford University Press.

Garcia, J. & Campbell, R. (1997) Asking the right questions. Chapter 2 in *The Organization of Maternity Care: A guide to evaluation* (eds R. Campbell & J. Garcia). Hale, Cheshire, Hochland & Hochland.

Garcia, J. & Garforth, S. (1989) Labour and delivery routines in English consultant maternity units. *Midwifery*, **5**(4) 155–62.

Garcia, J., Kilpatrick, R. & Richards, M. (1990) *The Politics of Maternity Care: Services for Childbearing women in Twentieth-Century Britain.* Oxford University Press.

Garcia, J. Renfrew, M. & Marchant, S. (1994) Postnatal home visiting by midwives. *Midwifery*, **10**(1) 40–3.

Gilliland, A.L. (1998) Commentary: nurses doulas and childbirth educators – working together for common goals. *Journal of Perinatal Education*, **7**(3) 18–24.

Ginzberg, E. (1998) The changing US Health Care Agenda. *Journal of the American Medical Association*, **279**(7) 501–4.

Gottlieb, B.H. (1981) Development and application of a classification scheme of informal helping behaviour. *Canadian Journal of Behavioral Science*, **10**, 105–15.

Graham, I.D. (1997) *Episiotomy: Challenging Obstetric Intervention.* Oxford, Blackwell Science.

Green, J. (1998) Postnatal depression or perinatal dysphoria? Findings from a longitudinal community based study using the Edinburgh Postnatal Depression Scale. *Journal of Reproductive and Infant Psychology*, **16**(2/3) 143–56.

Green, J.M., Coupland, V.A. & Kitzinger, J.V. (1990) Expectations experiences and psychological outcomes of childbirth: A prospective study of 825 women. *Birth*, **17**, 15–24.

Ham, C. (1992) *Health Policy in Britain*, 3rd edn. London, Macmillan.

Ham, C., Robinson, R., Benzeval, M. (1990) *Health Check: Health care reforms in an international context.* London, Kings Fund Institute.

Hamilton, M. (1998) Patterns of postnatal visiting: the views of women and midwives. *British Journal of Midwifery*, **6**(1) 15–18.

Hansen, L.B. & Jacob, E. (1992) Intergenerational support during the transition to parenthood – issues for new parents and grandparents. *Families in Society* – the journal of contemporary human services, **73**(8) 471–9.

Hanson, J. (2000a) Why Hire a Doula? *Pregnancy Today* http://pregnancy today.co

Hanson, J. (2000b) Mother-friendly trends. *Pregnancy Today* http://pregnancy today.co

Harcombe, J. (1999) Power and political power positions in maternity care. *British Journal of Midwifery*, **7**(2) 78–82.

Hardy, M. & Mulhall, A. (1994) *Nursing Research Theory and Practice.* London, Chapman & Hall.

Hart, A., Pankhurst, F.L. & Sommerville, F. (1999) An evaluation of team midwifery. *British Journal of Midwifery*, **7**(9) 573–8.

Havighurst, C.C., Helms, R.B., Bladen, C. & Pauly, M.V. (1988) *American Health Care: What are the lessons for Britain?* London, IEA Health Unit.

Hawkins, P. & Shohet, R. (1989) *Supervision in the Helping Professions: an individual, group and organizational approach.* Milton Keynes, Open University Press.

HEBS (1995) *The Breastfeeding Facts Pack.* Edinburgh, Health Education Board for Scotland.

Heginbotham, C. (1994) Consumer Groups Section 3.4 241 in *NHS Handbook* (ed P. Merry), 9th Edition. Tunbridge Wells, NAHAT/JMH Publishing.

Helms, R.B. & Bladen, C. (1988) Creating incentives for competition. Part 1 in *American Health Care: What are the lessons for Britain?* (C.C. Havighurst, R.B. Helms, C. Blanden & M.V. Pauly). London, IEA Health Unit.

Herbert, P. (1994) Support of first-time mothers in the three months after birth. *Nursing Times,* **90**(24) 36–7.

Hiddinga, A. (1993) Dutch Obstetric Science: Emergence, Growth, and Present Situation, pp. 45–76. In *Successful Home Birth and Midwifery: The Dutch Model* (ed. M.E. Van der Abraham). London, Bergin & Garvey.

Hildingsson, I. & Häggström, T. (1999) Midwives, lived experiences of being supportive to prospective mothers/parents during pregnancy. *Midwifery,* **15**(2) 82–91.

Hillhouse, J.J. & Adler, C.M. (1997) Investigating stress effect patterns in hospital staff nurses: results of a cluster analysis. *Social Science & Medicine,* **45**(12) 1781–8.

Hingley, P. & Marks, R. (1991) A stressful occupation. *Nursing Times,* **87**(25) 63–6.

Hingstman, L. (1994) Primary care obstetrics and perinatal health in the Netherlands. *Journal of Nurse-Midwifery,* **39**(6) 379–86.

Hochschild, A. (1979) Emotion work, feeling rules and social structure. *American Journal of Sociology,* **85**, 551–75.

Hodnett, E. (1997) Commentary: Are nurses effective providers of labour support? Can they be? Should they be? *Birth,* June, **24**(2) 78–80.

Hodnett E.D. (2000a) Support during pregnancy for women at increased risk. *The Cochrane Database of Systematic Reviews,* issue 1. The Cochrane Library, Copyright The Cochrane Collaboration.

Hodnett, E.D. (2000b) Continuity of caregivers for care during pregnancy and childbirth. *The Cochrane Database of Systematic Reviews,* issue 1. The Cochrane Library, Copyright The Cochrane Collaboration.

Hodnett, E.D. (2000c) *Caregiver support for women during childbirth.* The Cochrane Database of Systematic Reviews, issue 1. The Cochrane Library, Copyright The Cochrane Collaboration.

Hodnett, E.D. & Osborn, R.W. (1989a) Effects of continuous intrapartum professional support on childbirth outcomes. *Research in Nursing & Health,* **12**, 289–297.

Hodnett, E.D. & Osborn, R.W. (1989b) A randomised trial of the effects of monitrice support during labor: Mothers' views two to four weeks postpartum. *Birth,* **16**(4) 177–83.

Hofmeyr, G.J., Nikodem, V.C., Wolman, W.L., Chalmers, B.E. & Kramer, T. (1991) Companionship to modify the clinical birth environment: effects on progress and perceptions of labour, and breastfeeding. *British Journal of Obstetrics and Gynaecology,* **98**, 756–64.

Hofmeyr, G.J. & Nikodem, V.C. (1994) Achieving mother and baby friendliness – the evidence for labour companions. Chapter 8, p.89 in *Baby Friendly Mother Friendly* (ed. S.F. Murray). London, Mosby.

Holden, J.M., Sagovsky, R. & Cox, J.L. (1989) Counselling in a general practice setting: controlled study of health visitor intervention in treatment of postnatal depression. *British Medical Journal,* **298**, 233–6.

Holroyd, E., Yin-King, L., Pui-Yuk, L.W., Kwok-Hong, F.Y. & Shuk-Lin B.L. (1997) Hong Kong Chinese women's perception of support from midwives during labour. *Midwifery,* **13**(2) 66–72.

House, G.S. (1981) *Work Stress and Social Support.* Reading, MA, Addison–Wesley.

House, J.S. & Kahn, R.L. (1985) Measures and concepts of social support. Chapter 5, pp. 83–108 in *Social Support and Health* (eds S. Cohen & S.L. Syme). Orlando, Academic Press.

House, J. Robbins, C. & Metzner, H. (1982) The association of social relationships and activities with mortality: prospective evidence from the Tecumseh Community Health Study. *American Journal of Epidemiology*, **116**, 123–40.

House, J.S., Landis, K.R. & Umberson, D. (1988) Social relationships and health. *Science*, **241**, 540–5.

Houston, M.J. (1981) Health service support for the breast feeding mother – an alternative approach? Research – A base for the future? *Conference Proceedings*. University of Edinburgh, Department of Nursing Studies.

Howell-White, S. (1997) Choosing a birth attendant: the influence of a woman's childbirth definition. *Social Science & Medicine*, **45**(6) 925–36.

Howie, P.W. (1985) Breast feeding – a new understanding. *Midwives Chronicle*, **98**(1170) 184–92.

Hundley, V.A., Cruickshank, F.M., Lang, G.D., Glazener, C.M.A., Milne, J.M., Turner, M., Blyth, D., Mollison, J. & Donaldson, C. (1994) Midwife managed delivery unit: a randomised controlled comparison with consultant led care. *British Medical Journal*, **309**(6966) 1400–4.

Hundley, V., Donaldson, C., Lang, G.D., Cruickshank, F.M., Glazener, C.M. A., Milne, J.M. & Mollison, J. (1995) Costs of intrapartum care in a midwife-managed delivery unit and a consultant led labour ward. *Midwifery*, **11**(3) 103–9.

Hundley, V.A., Milne, J.M., Glazener, C.M. & Mollison, J. (1997) Satisfaction and the three Cs: continuity, choice and control. Women's views from a randomised controlled trial of midwife-led care. *British Journal of Obstetrics and Gynaecology*, **104**(11) 1273–80.

Hunter, D.J. (1993) To Market! To Market! A new dawn for community health care? *Health and Social Care in the Community*, **1**(1) 3–10.

Hupcey, J.E. (1998) Clarifying the social support theory-research linkage. *Journal of Advanced Nursing*, **27**(6) 1231–41.

Ip, W.Y. (2000) Relationships between partner's support during labour and maternal outcomes. *Journal of Clinical Nursing*, **9**(2) 265–72.

Isherwood, K. (1988) Friend or watchdog? . . . duties of a supervisor of midwives. *Nursing Times*, **84**(24) 15–21.

Isherwood, K. (1989) Independent Midwifery in the U.K *Midwife Health Visitor and Community Nurse*, **25**(7) 307–9.

Jabaaij, L. & Meijer, W. (1996) Home births in the Netherlands: midwifery-related factors of influence. *Midwifery*, **12**(3) 129 35.

Jackson, C. & Mander, R. (1995) History or herstory: the decline and fall of the midwife? *British Journal of Midwifery*, **3**, 5279–83.

Jeffery, P., Jeffery, R. & Lyon, A. (1989) *Labour Pains and Labour Power: women and childbearing in India*. London, Zed Books.

Jenkins, R. (1995) *The Law and the Midwife*. Oxford, Blackwell.

Johnson, R. (1996) Enabling midwives to practise better. Chapter 7, p.90 in *Supervision of Midwives* (ed. M. Kirkham). Hale, Books for Midwives Press.

Johnson, T. (1995) Governmentality and the institutionalisation of expertise. Chapter 1, pp. 7–23 in *Health Professions and the State in Europe* (eds T. Johnson, G. Larkin & M. Saks). London, Routledge.

Jordan, B. (1978) *Birth in Four Cultures: A crosscultural investigation of childbirth in Yucatan, Holland, Sweden and the United States*. Vermont, Eden Press.

Kaczorowski, J., Levitt, C., Hanvey, L., Avard, D. & Change, G. (1998) A national survey of use of obstetric procedures and technologies in Canadian hospitals: routine or based on existing evidence? *Birth*, **25**(1) 11–18.

Kahn, R.L. & Antonucci, T.C. (1980) Convoys over the life course: Attachment roles and social support, pp. 253–86 in *Life Span Development and Behavior* (eds P.B. Baltes & O. Brim). New York, Academic Press.

Kaufman, K. & McDonald, H. (1988) A retrospective evaluation of a model of midwifery care. *Birth*, **15**(2) 95–9.

Keirse, M.J.N.C., Enkin, M. & Lumley, J. (1989) Social and professional support during childbirth. Chapter 49 in *Effective Care in Pregnancy and Childbirth* (eds I. Chalmers, M. Enkin & M.J.N.C. Keirse) vol. 2. Oxford University Press.

Keirse, M.J. (1993) A final comment ... managing the uterus, the woman, or whom?. *Birth*, **20**(3) 159–61.

Kennell, J. Klaus, M., McGrath, S., Robertson, S. & Hinkley, C. (1991) Continuous emotional support during labour in a US hospital. *Journal of the American Medical Association*, **265**(17) 2197–2201.

Kirkham, M. (1986) A feminist perspective in midwifery. Chapter 3 in *Feminist Practice in Women's Health Care* (ed. C. Webb). Chichester, John Wiley.

Kirkham, M. (1989) Midwives and information giving during labour. In *Midwives Research and Childbirth* (S. Robinson & A. Thomson), vol. 1. London, Chapman & Hall.

Kirkham, M. (1999) The culture of midwifery in the National Health Service in England. *Journal of Advanced Nursing*, **30**(3) 732–9.

Kirkham, M. (2000) Midwives' support needs as childbirth changes. *Journal of Advanced Nursing*, **32**(2) 465–72.

Kistin, N., Abramson, R. & Dublin, P. (1994) Effect of peer counselors on breastfeeding initiation, exclusivity, and duration among low-income urban women. *Journal of Human Lactation*, **10**(1) 11–15.

Kitzinger, J.V. (1992) Counteracting, not re-enacting, the violation of women's bodies: the challenge for perinatal caregivers. *Birth*, **19**(4) 219–20.

Kitzinger, S. (1978) *Women as Mothers*. Glasgow, Fontana/Collins.

Kitzinger, S. (1998) Sheila Kitzinger's letter from Europe: the cesarean epidemic in Great Britain (letter). *Birth*, **25**(1) 56–8.

Kitzinger, S. (2000) Being there. *The Guardian*, 18 January, 4–5.

Klaus, M.H. & Kennell, J.H. (1976) *Maternal-infant Bonding*. St Louis, C.V. Mosby.

Klaus, M.H. & Kennell, J.H. (1997) The doula: an essential ingredient of childbirth rediscovered. *Acta Paediatrica*, **86**(10) 1034–6.

Klaus, M.H., Kennell, J.H. & Klaus, P.H. (1993) *Mothering the Mother: How a doula can help you have a shorter easier and healthier birth*. Reading, Mass, Addison Wesley.

Klaus, M.H., Kennell, J.H., Robertson, S.S. & Sosa, R. (1986) Effects of social support during parturition on maternal and infant morbidity. *British Medical Journal*, **293**, 585–7.

Klein, M.C. (1997) Letter: One-to-one nurse support in labour. *Birth*, **24**(4) 270–1.

Lackner, S., Goldengerg, S., Arrizza, G. & T Josvold, I. (1994) The contingency of social support. *Qualitative Health Research*, **4**, 224–43.

Lalonde Report (1974) *A new perspective on the health of Canadians*. Ottawa, Ministry of National Health and Welfare.

Langer, A., Campero, L., Garcia, C. & Reynoso, S. (1998) Effects of psychosocial support during labour and childbirth on breastfeeding, medical interventions and mothers' wellbeing in a Mexican public hospital: a randomised clinical trial. *British Journal of Obstetrics & Gynaecology*, **105**(10) 1056–63.

Langer, A., Farnot, U., Garcia, C., Barros, F., Victora, C., Belizan, J.M. & Villar, J. (1996) The Latin American trial of psychosocial support during pregnancy: effects on mother's wellbeing and satisfaction. *Social Science and Medicine*, **42**(11) 1589–97.

Langford, C.P.H., Bowsher, J., Maloney, J.P. & Lillis, P.P. (1997) Social support: a conceptual analysis. *Journal of Advanced Nursing*, **25**(1) 95–100.

Larkin, G. (1994) State control and the health professions in the UK: historical perspectives. Chapter 3, pp.45–54 in *Health Professions and the State in Europe* (eds T. Johnson, G. Larkin & M. Saks). London, Routledge.

Laughlin, S. & Black, D. (1995) *Poverty and Health: Tools for change*. Birmingham, Public Health Alliance.

Lauwers, J. & Shinskie, D. (2000) *Counseling the Nursing Mother: a lactation consultant's guide*, 3rd edn. Sudbury, Mass, Jones & Bartlett.

Lavender, T. & Walkinshaw, S.A. (1998) Can midwives reduce postpartum psychological morbidity? A randomized trial. *Birth*, **25**(4) 215–19.

Lavender, T. & Walkinshaw, S.A. & Walton, I. (1999) A prospective study of women's views of factors contributing to a positive birth experience. *Midwifery*, **15**(1) 40–6.

Lazarus, R. (1966) *Psychological Stress and the Coping Process*. McGraw-Hill, New York.

Leap, N. (1997) Making sense of 'horizontal violence' in midwifery. *British Journal of Midwifery*, **5**(11) 689.

Leavy, R.L. (1983) Social support and psychological disorder: a review. *Journal of Community Psychology*, **11**, 3–21.

Lederberg, M.S. (1998) Staff support groups for high stress medical environments. *International Journal of Group Psychotherapy*, **48**(2) 275–304.

Levitt, R., Wall, A. & Appleby, J. (1995) *The Reorganised National Health Service*, 5th edn. London, Chapman & Hall.

Lewis, C. (1986) *Becoming a Father*. Milton Keynes, Open University Press.

Lewis, P. (1996) The death of Changing Childbirth *Modern Midwife*, **5**(5) 32–3.

Lewison, H. (1996) Supervision as a public service. Chapter 5, pp.72–83 in *Supervision of Midwives* (ed. M. Kirkham). Hale, Books for Midwives Press.

Loudon, I. (1992) *Death in Childbirth: An international study of maternal care and maternal mortality 1800–1950*. Oxford, Clarendon Press.

Lovell, A. (1983) Women's reactions to late miscarriage, stillbirth and perinatal death. *Health Visitor*, **56**, 325–7.

Lubic, R.W. (1979) *Barriers and Conflict in Maternity Care Innovation*. New York City, Maternity Center Association.

Lundgren, I. & Dahlberg, K. (1998) Women's experience of pain during childbirth. *Midwifery*, **14**(2) 105–10.

MacArthur, C. (1999) What does postnatal care do for women's health? *The Lancet*, **353**(9150) 343–4.

MacArthur, C., Lewis, M. & Knox, E.G. (1991) *Health after Childbirth*. London, The Stationery Office.

Macdonald, A.M. (1981) *Chambers Twentieth Century Dictionary*. Edinburgh, Chambers Ltd.

Mackin, P. & Sinclair, M. (1998) Labour ward midwives' perceptions of stress. *Journal of Advanced Nursing*, **27**(5) 986–91.

MacMillan, M. (1998) *Men at Birth*. London, Royal College of Midwives.

Madi, B.C., Sandall, J., Bennett, V.R. & MacLeod, C. (1999) Effects of female relative support in labour: a randomised controlled trial. *Birth*, **26**(1) 4–8.

Mainord, M. (1997) Doulas: aids or opportunists? *Tennessee Nurse*, **60**(3) 21.

Mander, R. (1992) See how they Learn: Experience as the basis of practice. *Nurse Education Today*, February, vol. 12, pp.11–18.

Mander, R. (1993) 'Who chooses the choices?' *Modern Midwife*, **3**(1) 23–5.

Mander, R. (1994) *Loss and Bereavement in Childbearing*. Oxford, Blackwell Scientific.

Mander, R. (1995) The relevance of the Dutch system of maternity care to the United Kingdom. *Journal of Advanced Nursing*, **22**(6) 1023–6.

Mander, R. (1996) The Childfree midwife: the significance of personal experience of childbearing. *Midwives*, **109**(1302) 186–8.

Mander, R. (1997) Choosing the choices in the USA: examples in the maternity area. *Journal of Advanced Nursing*, **25**(6) 1192–7.

Mander, R. (1998) *Pain in Childbearing and its Control*. Oxford, Blackwell Scientific.

Mander, R. (1999a) The death of a mother – a proposed research project. *RCM Midwives Journal*, **2**(1) 24–5.

Mander, R. (1999b) Preliminary report: A study of the midwife's experience of the death of a mother. *RCM Midwives Journal*, **2**(11) 346–9.

Maresh, M. (1999) Auditing care. Chapter 9, pp. 137–52 in *Community-based Maternity Care* (eds G. Marsh & M. Renfrew). Oxford General Practice Series, Oxford University Press.

Marland, H. (1993) The '*burgerlijke*' midwife: the *stadsvroedvrouw* of eighteenth century

Holland. Chapter 10, p.192 in *The Art of Midwifery: Early modern midwives in Europe* (ed. H. Marland). London, Routledge.

Marsh, J. & Sargent, E. (1991) Factors affecting the duration of postnatal visits. *Midwifery*, **7**(4) 177–82.

Martin-Hirsch, J. & Wright, G. (1998) The development of a quality model: measuring effective midwifery services (MEMS). *International Journal of Health Care Quality Assurance*, **11**(2–3) 50–7.

Maslach, C. (1976) Burned Out. *Human Behavior*, **5**, 16–22.

Maslach, C. (1981) *Burnout: the Cost of Caring*. Prentice Hall, Englewood Cliffs, New Jersey.

Mason, J. (2000) Letter: Midwives 'verging on the sadistic'. *British Journal of Midwifery*, **8**(4) 247.

Matrunola, P. (1996) Is there a relationship between job satisfaction and absenteeism? *Journal of Advanced Nursing*, **23**(4) 827–34.

Matthews, S., Stansfeld, S. & Power, C. (1999) Social support at age 33: the influence of gender, employment and social class. *Social Science & Medicine*, **49**(1) 133–42.

Maynard, A. (1994) Can competition enhance efficiency in health care? Lessons from the reform of the UK national health service. *Social Science & Medicine*, **39**(10) 1433–45.

McCandlish, R. (1999) *Caesarean Epidemic*. Departmental Seminar. Department of Nursing Studies, University of Edinburgh.

McConnell, E.A. (2000) Nursing Publications outside the United States. *Journal of Nursing Scholarship*, **32**(1) 87–92.

McCourt, C. & Page, L. (1996) *Report on the evaluation of one-to-one midwifery*. London, Centre for Midwifery Practice.

McCourt, C., Page, L., Hewison, J. & Vail, A. (1998) Evaluation of one-to-one midwifery: women's responses to care. *Birth*, **25**(2) 73–80.

McCullough, P.G. & Rutenberg, S.K. (1989) Launching children and moving on. Chapter 13, pp.285–309 in *The Changing Family Life Cycle* (eds B. Caster & M. McGoldrick) 2nd edn. Boston, Allyn & Bacon.

McEwen, B.S. (1998) Protective and damaging effects of stress mediators. *New England Journal of Medicine*, **338**(3) 171–9.

McGinley, M., Turnbull, D., Fyvie, H., Johnstone, I. & MacLennan, B. (1995) Midwifery development unit at Glasgow Royal Maternity Hospital. *British Journal of Midwifery*, **3**(7) 362–71.

McHaffie, H. (1996) Supporting families with a very low birthweight baby. Chapter 11, pp.238–63 in *Midwives Research and Childbirth* (eds S. Robinson & A.M. Thomson) vol. 4. London, Chapman & Hall.

McKee, I.H. (1984) Community antenatal care: The Sighthill community antenatal scheme. Chapter 5 in *Pregnancy Care for the 1980s* (eds L. Zander & G. Chamberlain). London, Royal Society of Medicine.

McNiven, P., Hodnett, E. & O'Brien-Pallas, E.L. (1992) Supporting women in labour. *Birth*, **19**(1) 3–8.

McSherry, R. & Haddock, J. (1999) Evidence based health care: its place within clinical governance. *British Journal of Nursing*, **8**(2) 113–7.

McVeigh, C.A. (1997) An Australian study of functional status after childbirth. *Midwifery*, **13**(4) 172–8.

Melzack, R. & Wall, P. (1991) *The Challenge of Pain*. London, Penguin.

Menzies, I.E.P. (1960) A case study in the functioning of social systems as a defence against anxiety. In *Threshold to Nursing* (ed. J. Macgure). London, Bell.

Metts, S., Geist, P. & Gray, J.L. (1994) The role of relationship characteristics in the provision and effectiveness of supportive messages among nursing professionals. Chapter 12, p.229 In *Communication of Social Support* (eds B.R. Burleson, T.L. Albrecht & I.G. Sarason). London, Sage.

MIDIRS (1996) *Support in Labour: informed choice for professionals*. York, Midwives Information & Resource Service & NHS Centre for Reviews and Dissemination.

MIDIRS (1997) *Informed Choice for Professionals*. York, Midwives Information & Research Service & NHS Centre for Reviews and Dissemination.

Miller, K. & Ray, E.B. (1994) Beyond the ties that bind us: Exploring the meaning of supportive messages and relationships. Chapter 11, pp. 215–28 in *Communication of social Support* (eds B.R. Barleson, T.L. Albrecht & I.G. Sarason). London, Sage.

MoH (1961) *Human relations in obstetrics*: Standing Maternity and Midwifery Advisory Committee: Ministry of Health. London, The Stationery Office.

Morgan, B.M., Bulpitt, C.J., Clifton, P. & Lewis, P.J. (1982) Analgesia and satisfaction in childbirth. *Lancet*, ii, 808–10.

Morgan, M., Fenwick, N., McKenzie, C. & Wolfe, C.D.A. (1998) Quality of midwifery-led care: assessing the effects of different models of continuity for women's satisfaction. *Quality in Health Care*, 7(?) 77–82.

Morison, S., Hauck, Y., Percival, P. & McMurray, A. (1998) Constructing a home birth environment through assuming control. *Midwifery*, 14(4) 233–41.

Munro, L., Rodwell, J. & Harding, L. (1998) Assessing occupational stress in psychiatric nurses using the full job strain model: the value of social support to nurses. *International Journal of Nursing Studies*, 35(6) 339–45.

Murray, S.F. & Pradenas, F.S. (1997) Caesarean birth trends in Chile 1986–1994. *Birth*, 24(4) 258–63.

NBS (1999) *Midwifery Supervision: maintaining and improving standards of practice and care*. Edinburgh, National Board for Nursing Midwifery and Health Visiting for Scotland.

NBS (undated) *Quality Assurance: Midwifery Supervision*. Edinburgh, National Board for Nursing Midwifery and Health Visiting for Scotland.

Neilson, J.P. (1999) The use of technology in maternity care. Chapter 13 in *Community-based Maternity Care* (eds G. Marsh & M. Renfrem). Oxford, Oxford University Press.

Neuberger, J. (1990) A consumer's view. In *The NHS Reforms: whatever happened to consumer choice*? (eds D.G., Green, J. Neuberger, L. Young & M.L., Burstall). London, IEA Health and Welfare Unit.

Neuffer, E. (1993) Clinton Care Plan: A policy primer in health care. *Boston Globe*, 26th August, p.1.

Newton, R.W. (1988) Psychosocial aspects of pregnancy: the scope for intervention. *Journal of Reproductive and Infant Psychology*, 6(1) 23–8.

Newton, R.W. & Hunt, L.P. (1984) Psychosocial stress in pregnancy and its relation to low birth weight. *British Medical Journal*, 288, 1191.

Niven, C.A. (1992) *Psychological Care for Families*. Oxford, Butterworth Heinemann.

Niven, C.A. (1994) Coping with labour pain: the midwife's role. In *Midwives Research and Childbirth* (eds S. Robinson & A.M. Thomson) vol. III. London, Chapman & Hall.

Nolan, M.L. & Hicks, C. (1997) Aims, processes and problems of antenatal education as identified by three groups of childbirth teachers. *Midwifery*, 13(4) 179–88.

Norbeck, J.S., Dejoseph, J.E. & Smith, R.T. (1996) A randomised trial of an empirically-derived social support intervention to prevent low birth weight among African American women. *Social Science and Medicine*, 43(6) 947–54.

O'Driscoll, K. & Meagher, D. (1986) *Active Management of Labour*, 2nd, edn. London, Baillière Tindall.

O'Driscoll, K., Meagher, D. & Boylan, P. (1993) *Active Management of Labour: The Dublin Experience*, 3rd edn. London, Mosby.

O'Driscoll, K. Stronge, J.M. & Minogue, M. (1973) Active management of labour. *British Medical Journal*, 3, 133–5.

O'Regan, M. (1998) Active management of labour: the Irish Way of Birth. *AIMS Journal*, 10(2) 1–7.

Oakley, A. (1988) Is social support good for the health of mothers and babies? *Journal of Reproductive and Infant Psychology*, 6(1) 3–21.

Oakley, A. (1992a) *Social Support and Motherhood*. Oxford, Blackwell.

Oakley, A. (1992b) Measuring the effectiveness of psychosocial interventions in pregnancy. *International Journal of Technology Assessment in Health Care*, 8(1) 129–38.

Oakley, A. (1992c) Commentary: The best research is that which breeds more. *Birth*, **19**(1) 8–9.

Oakley, A., Rajan, L. & Grant, A. (1990) Social support and pregnancy outcome (SSPO), *British Journal of Obstetrics and Gynaecology*, **97**, 155–62.

Odent, M. (1996) Why labouring women don't need 'support'. *Mothering*, **80**, Autumn, 47–51.

Odent, M. (2000) Being there. *The Guardian*, January 18, 4–5.

Olds, S.B., London, M.L. & Ladewig, P.W. (1996) *Maternal Newborn Nursing: a family centred approach*. Menlo Park, Addison-Wesley.

Oliver, S., Rajan, L., Turner, H., Oakley, A., Entwistle, V., Watt, I., Sheldon, T.A. & Rosser, J. (1996) Informed choice for users of health services: views on ultrasonography leaflets of women in early pregnancy, midwives, and ultrasonographers. *British Medical Journal*, **313**(7067) 1251–3.

ONS (1996) Office for National Statistics *Population and Health Monitor DH3 96/1*. London, The Stationery Office.

ONS (1997) *Infant Feeding 1995*. Office for National Statistics. London, The Stationery Office.

Orth-Gomer, K. & Unden, L.A. (1987) The measurement of social support in population surveys. *Social Science and Medicine*, **24**(1) 83–94.

Page, L. (1996) The backlash against evidence-based care. *Birth*, **23**(4) 191–2.

Page, L. (1997) The backlash against evidence-based care. *MIDIRS Midwifery Digest*, **7**(2) 146–7.

Page, L., McCourt, C., Beake, S., Vail, A. & Hewison, J. (1999) Clinical interventions and outcomes of one-to-one midwifery practice. *Journal of Public Health Medicine*, **21**(3) 243–8.

Palmer, G. (1993) *The Politics of Breastfeeding*. London, Pandora.

Palmer, G. & Kemp, S. (1994) Breastfeeding promotion and the role of the professional midwife. Chapter 1 in *Baby friendly mother friendly* (ed. S.F. Murray) pp. 1–23. St Louis, Mosby.

Paton, C. (1995) *Competition and Planning in the NHS: the danger of unplanned markets*. London, Chapman & Hall.

Paton, C. (1996) *Health Policy and Management: the healthcare agenda in the British political context*. London, Chapman & Hall.

Pauly, M.V. (1988) Efficiency equity and costs in the US health care system. Part 2 in *American Health Care: What are the lessons for Britain*? (eds C.C. Havighurst, R.B., Helms, C. Bladen & M.V. Pauly) Paper No. 5, London, IEA Health Unit.

Piotrowski, K. (1997) First stage of labour. Chapter 17, p.352 in *Maternity and Woman's Health Care*, (eds D.L. Loudermilk, S.E. Perry & I.M. Bobak) 6th edn. St Louis, Mosby.

Playle, J.F. & Mullarkey, K. (1998) Parallel process in clinical supervision: enhancing learning and providing support. *Nurse Education Today*, **18**(7) 558–66.

Podkolinski, J. (1998) Women's experience of postnatal support. Chapter 11, p.205 in *Psychological Perspectives on Pregnancy and Childbirth* (ed. S. Clement). Edinburgh, Churchill Livingstone.

Poole, M. (1999) The effect of selective visiting on maternal anxiety. *British Journal of Midwifery*, **7**(3), 144–9.

Porreco, R.P. & Thorp, J.A. (1996) The cesarean birth epidemic: trends, causes, and solutions. *American Journal of Obstetrics & Gynecology*, **175**(2) 369–74.

Power, M.J., Champion, L.A. & Aris, S.J. (1988) The development of a measure of social support: the significant others (SOS) scale. *British Journal of Clinical Psychology*, **27**, 349–58.

Rådestad, I., Nordin, C., Steineck, G. & Sjögren, B. (1996) Stillbirth is no longer managed as a nonevent: A nationwide study in Sweden. *Birth*, **23**(4) 209–15.

Rajan, L. & Oakley, A. (1993) No pills for heartache: the importance of social support for women who suffer pregnancy loss. *Journal of Reproductive and Infant Psychology*, **11**(2) 75–88.

Raphael, D. (1973) *The Tender Gift: Breastfeeding*. Englewood Cliffs, NJ, Prentice-Hall.

Raphael, D. (1981) The midwife as doula: a guide to mothering the mother. *Journal of Nurse-Midwifery*, **26**, 13–15.

Raphael, D. (1988) New patterns in doula client relations … doula, the neighbour who walks across the street and helps after the baby is born. *Midwife, Health Visitor & Community Nurse*, **24**(9) 376, 378–9.

Raphael-Leff, J. (1991) *Psychological Processes of Childbearing*, London, Chapman & Hall.

Ray, K.L. & Hodnett, E.D. (2000) Caregiver support for postpartum depression *The Cochrane Database of Systematic Reviews*, Cochrane Pregnancy and Childbirth Group. The Cochrane Library, The Cochrane Collaboration (issue 1).

Rees, C. (1997) *An Introduction to Research for Midwives*. Hale, Hochland & Hochland.

Reid, M. (1997) A randomised controlled trial of two interventions to provide social support. *British Journal of Midwifery*, **5**(10) 610, 612.

Reid, L. Hillan, E. & Mcguire, M. (1997) Midwives and woman-centred care. The challenge of negotiating the maze of woman-centred care in Scotland. *British Journal of Midwifery*, **5**(10) 602, 604–6.

Reid, M., Lang, G., Prigg, S., Murray, G., Glazener, C., Mackenzie, J. & Connery, L. (1999) *Final Report: A two centred randomised controlled trial of two forms of postnatal support*. University of Glasgow.

Relyea, M. (1992) The rebirth of midwifery in Canada – an historical perspective. *Midwifery*, **8**(4) 159–69.

Rennie, A-M., Hundley, V., Gurney, E. & Graham, W. (1998) Women's priorities for care before and after delivery. *British Journal of Midwifery*, **6**(7) 434–8.

Revans, R.W. (1964) *Standards for Morale: cause and effect in hospitals*. The Nuffield Provincial Hospitals Trust, Oxford University Press.

Richards, M.P.M. (1982) The trouble with choice in childbirth. *Birth*, **9**(4) 253–60.

Richards, M.P.M. (2000) Commentary: Assessing women's well-being and social and emotional needs in pregnancy and the post partum period. *Birth*, **27**(2) 102–3.

Rini, C.K., Dunkel-Schetter, C. Wadhwa, P.D. & Sandman, C.A. (1999) Psychological adaptation and birth outcomes: the role of personal resources, stress and sociocultural context in pregnancy. *Health Psychology*, **18**(4) 333–45.

Riordan, J. & Auerbach, K.G. (2000) *Clinical Lactation: A visual guide*. Sudbury, Mass., Jones & Bartlett.

Roberts, J. (1996) Changing Childbirth–Choices and Costs. *MIDIRS Midwifery Digest*, **6**(3) 261–3.

Robertson, A. (1997) *The Midwife Companion – the art of support during birth*. Camber, Ace Graphics.

Robinson, J. (1998) What do doulas do? *AIMS Journal*, **10**(3) 20.

Robinson, J. (1999) Birth companions and postnatal depression. *AIMS Journal*, **11**(1) 16.

Robinson, S. (1990) Maintaining the independence of the midwifery professions: a continuing struggle. In *The Politics of Maternity care: Services for Childbearing women in Twentieth-Century Britain* (eds J. Garcia, R. Kilpatrich & M. Richards), Oxford University Press.

Robinson, S., Golden, J. & Bradley, S. (1983) *A study of the role and responsibilities of the midwife*. Nursing Education Research Unit Report 1 University of London, Kings College.

Rothwell, H. (1996) Changing childbirth changing nothing. *Midwives*, **109**(1306) 291–4.

Rowley, M.J. Hensley, M.J., Brinsmead, M.W. & Wlodarczyk, J.H. (1995) Continuity of care by a midwife team versus routine care during pregnancy and birth: a randomised trial. *Medical Journal of Australia*, **163**(6) 289–93.

Ruble, D.N. Fleming, A.S., Hackel, L.S. & Stangor, C. (1988) Changes in the marital relationship during the transition to first time motherhood. *Journal of Personality and Social Psychology*, **55**(1) 78–87.

Sackett, D., Rosenburg, W., Gray, J., Haynes, B. & Richardson, W.S. (1996) Evidence based medicine: what it is and what it isn't. *British Medical Journal*, **312** (7023) 71–2.

Sagady, M. (1997) Letter: One-to-one nurse support in labour. *Birth*, **24**(4) 271–2.

Saltman, R.B. (1997) Equity and distributive justice in European health care reform. *International Journal of Health Services*, **27**(3) 443–53.

Sandall, J. (1997) Midwives' burnout and continuity of care. *British Journal of Midwifery*, **5**(2) 106–11.

Sandall, J. (1998) Occupational burnout in midwives: new ways of working and the relationship between organizational factors and psychological health and wellbeing. *Risk Decision and Policy*, **3**(3) 213–32.

Sandall, J. (1999) Team midwifery and burnout in midwives in the UK: practical lessons from a national study. *MIDIRS Midwifery Digest*, **9**(2), 147–52.

Sarason, I.G. Sarason, B.R. & Pierce, G.R. (1990) Relationship specific social support: towards a model for the analysis of supportive interactions. Chapter 5, p.91 in *Communication of Social Support*, (eds B.R. Barleson, T.L. Albrecht & I.G. Sarason). London, Sage.

Scally, G. & Donaldson, L. (1998) Looking forward clinical governance and the drive for quality improvement in the new NHS in England. *British Medical Journal*, **317**(7150) 61–5.

Schoon, L. (1995) *De gynaecologie als belichaming van vrouwen: Verloskunde en gynaecologie 1840–1920*. Zutphen: Walburg Press.

Schott, J. & Henley, A. (1996) *Culture, Religion and Childbearing in a Multiracial Society: A handbook for health professionals*. Oxford, Butterworth Heinemann.

Schumaker, S.A. & Brownell, A. (1984) Toward a theory of social support: closing conceptual gaps. *Journal of Social Issues*, **40**(4) 11–36.

Schwarzer, R. & Leppin, A. (1990) *A meta analysis of social support research*. Unpublished paper, Free University of Berlin.

Scott, G. & Niven, C. (1996) Pregnancy: a bio-psycho-social event. In *Conception, Pregnancy and Birth* (eds C.A. Niven & A. Walker). Oxford, Butterworth Heinemann.

Scott, K.D., Berkowitz, G. & Klaus, M.A. (1999) A comparison of intermittent and continuous support during labor: a meta-analysis. *American Journal of Obstetrics and Gynecology*, **180**(5) 1054–9.

Seedhouse, D. (1995) Introduction: the logic of Health Reform. In *Reforming Health Care: The philosophy and practice of international health reform* (ed. D. Seedhouse). London, Wiley.

Séguin, L., Therrien, R., Champagne, F. & Larouche, D. (1989) T components of women's satisfaction with maternity care. *Birth*, **16**(3) 109–13.

Selman, P. & Haines, E. (1999) The social context of maternity care. Chapter 7 in *Community-based midwifery care* (eds G. Marsh & M.J. Renfrew). Oxford, Medical Publications.

SELMG (1994) Independent means. *Nursing Times*, **90**(4) 40–42.

Selye, H. (1936) Syndrome produced by diverse nocuous agents. *Nature*, **138**, 132.

Selye, H. (1956) *The Stress of Life*, 2nd edn. New York, McGraw-Hill.

Senden, I.P.M., van der Wettering, M.D., Eskes, A.B., Bierkens, P.B., Laube, D.W. & Pitkin, M.D. (1988) Labour pain: a comparison of parturients in a Dutch and an American teaching hospital. *Obstetrics & Gynecology*, **71**(4) 451–3.

Sheahan, D. (1972) The Game of the Name: Nurse Professional and Nurse Technician. *Nursing Outlook*, **20**(7) 440–5.

Shennan, C. (1996) Midwives' perceptions of the role of the supervisor of midwives. Chapter 12, p.168 in *Supervision of Midwives* (ed. M. Kirkham). Hale, Books for Midwives Press.

Shields, D. (1978) Nursing care in labour and patient satisfaction. *Journal of Advanced Nursing*, **3**(6) 535–50.

Shields, N., Turnbull, D., Reid, M., Holmes, A., McGinley, M. & Smith, L. (1998) Satisfaction with midwife-managed care in different time periods: a randomised controlled trial of 1299 women. *Midwifery*, **14**(2) 85–93.

Siddiqui, J. (1999) The therapeutic relationship in midwifery. *British Journal of Midwifery*, **7**(2) 111–14.

Sideris, M. (1996) *English-Greek/Greek-English Dictionary*. M. Sideris, Athens

Sidney, D. (1999) The burden of choice: reflections on independent practice. *MIDIRS Midwifery Digest*, **9**(1) 59–61.

Simkin, P. (1992) Just another day in a woman's life? Nature and consistency of women's long-term memories of their first birth experiences ... part 2. *Birth*, **19**(2) 64–81.

Simkin, P. & Way, K. (1998) Doulas of North America Position Paper: *The doula's contribution to modern maternity care*. http://www.dona.com/positionpapers.html/

Simkin, P. & Ancheta, R. (2000) *The Labor Progress Handbook*. Oxford, Blackwell Science.

Sleep, J. (1984) The West Berkshire Episiotomy Trial. In *Research and the Midwife conference proceedings* (eds A. Thomson & S. Robinson). Manchester University.

Sleutel, M.R. (2000) Intrapartum nursing care: a case study of supportive interventions and ethical conflicts. *Birth*, **27**(1) 38–45.

Smale, M. (1998) Working with breastfeeding mothers: the psychosocial context. Chapter 10 in *Psychological Perspectives on Pregnancy and Childbirth* (ed. S. Clement) pp. 183–204. Edinburgh, Churchill Livingstone.

Soderstrom, N.B., Chamberlain, M., Kaitell, C. & Stewart, P.J. (1990) Midwifery in Ontario: a survey of interest in services. *Birth*, **17**(3) 139–45.

Somers-Smith, M. (1999) A place for the partner? Expectations and experiences of support during childbirth. *Midwifery*, **15**(2) 101–8.

Soobader, M. & Leclere, F.B. (1999) Aggregation and the measurement of income inequality: effects on morbidity. *Social Science & Medicine*, **48**(6) 733–44.

Sosa, R., Kennell, J., Klaus, M., Robertson, S. & Urruttia, J. (1980) The effect of a supportive companion on perinatal problems, length of labour and mother-infant interaction. *New England Journal of Medicine*, **303**(11) 597–600.

Spencer, B., Thomas, H. & Morris, J. (1989) A randomised controlled trial of the provision of a social support service during pregnancy: the South Manchester Family Worker Project. *British Journal of Obstetrics and Gynaecology*, **96**, 3.

Spiby, H., Henderson, B., Slade, P., Escott, D. & Fraser, R.B. (1999) Strategies for coping with labour: does antenatal education translate into practice? *Journal of Advanced Nursing*, **29**(2) 388–94.

Spitzer, A., Bar-Tal, Y. & Golander, H. (1995) Social support: how does it really work? *Journal of Advanced Nursing*, **22**, 850–54.

Staines, C. (1986) Community co-operation in pre-natal care. In *Quest for Quality* (ed. Nursing Studies Association). University of Edinburgh.

Stansfield, P. (1997) An ancient tradition revived. *New Generation*, **16**(3) Sept, 8. (*MIDIRS Midwifery Digest*, **8**(1) 65–6.

Stapleton, H., Duerden, J. & Kirkham, M. (1998) *Evaluation of the impact of the supervision of midwives on professional practice and the quality of midwifery care*. University of Sheffield & English National Board for Nursing Midwifery and Health Visiting.

Stavropoulos, D.N. & Hornby, A.S. (1977) *Oxford English-Greek Learner's Dictionary*. Oxford University Press.

Stoter, D.J. (1997) *Staff Support in Health Care*. Oxford, Blackwell Science.

Sudbery, J. & Bradley, J. (1996) Staff support in organisations providing therapeutic Care. *Journal of Social Work Practice*, **26**(4) 648.

Sullivan-Lyons, J. (1998) Men becoming fathers: 'Sometimes I wonder how I'll cope'. Chapter 12 in *Psychological Perspectives on Pregnancy and Childbirth* (ed. S. Clement). Edinburgh, Churchill Livingstone.

Symon, A. (1996) Midwives and professional status. *British Journal of Midwifery*, **4**(10) 543–50.

Tarkka, M.-T. & Paunonen, M. (1996) Social support and its impact on mothers' experiences of childbirth. *Journal of Advanced Nursing*, **23**(1) 70–75.

van Teijlingen, E. (1994) *A social or medical model of childbirth? Comparing the arguments in Grampian (Scotland) and the Netherlands*. Unpublished PhD thesis, University of Aberdeen.

van Teijlingen, E. & McCaffery, P. (1987) The Profession of midwife in the Netherlands. *Midwifery*, **3**(3) 178–86.

van Teijlingen, E. & van der Hulst, L. (1995) Midwifery in the Netherlands: More than a semi profession? Chapter 11, pp.179–86 in *Health Professions in Europe* (eds T. Johnson, G. Larkin & M. Saks). London, Routledge.

Tew, M. (1995) *Safer Childbirth? – A critical history of maternity care*, 2nd edn. London, Chapman & Hall.

Thoits, P.A. (1982) Conceptual methodological and theoretical problems in studying social support as a buffer against life stress. *Journal of Health and Social Behavior*, **23**, 145–59.

Thomson, A.M. (1989) Why don't women breast feed? Chapter 11 in *Midwives Research and Childbirth* (eds S. Robinson & A.M. Thomson) pp.215–41. London, Chapman & Hall.

Thomson, A.M. (1993) Pushing techniques in the second stage of labour. *Journal of Advanced Nursing*, **18**(2) Feb, 171–7.

Tilden, V.P. & Gaylen, R.D. (1987) Cost and conflict: The darker side of social support. *Western Journal of Nursing Research*, **9**(1) 9–18.

Tinkler, A. & Quinney, D. (1998) Team midwifery: the influence of the midwife-woman relationship on women's experiences and perceptions of maternity care. *Journal of Advanced Nursing*, **28**(1) 30–35.

Todd, C.J., Farquhar, M.C., Camilleri-Ferrante, C. (1998) Team Midwifery: the views and job satisfaction of midwives. *Midwifery*, **14**(4) 214–24.

Tom, S.A. (1982) Political midwifery. *Journal of Nurse Midwifery*, **27**(3) 19–20.

Towler, J. & Bramall, J. (1986). *Midwives in History and Society*. London, Croom Helm.

Troll, L.E. (1983) Grandparents the family watchdogs. Chapter 5, pp.63–74 in *Family Relationships in Later Life* (ed. T.H. Brubacker). Beverly Hills Sage.

Turnbull, D., Homes, A., Shields, N., Cheyne, H., Twaddle, S., Gilmour, W.H., McCinley, M., Reid, M., Johnstone, I., Greer, I., McIlwaine, G. & Lunan, C.B. (1996) Randomised controlled trial of efficacy of midwife-managed care. *Lancet*, **348**(9022) 213–18.

Turnbull, D., Shields, N., McGinley, M., Holmes, A., Cheyne, H., Reid, M., Young, D. & Harper Gilmour, W. (1999) Can midwife-managed units improve continuity of care? *British Journal of Midwifery*, **7**(8) 499–503.

Twaddle, S. & Young, D. (1999) The economics of maternity care. Chapter 8, pp.119–136 in *Community-based Maternity Care* (eds M.J. Refrew & G. Marsh). Oxford University Press.

UKCC (1999) *Midwives Rules*. London, United Kingdom Central Council for Nursing, Midwifery and Health.

Umberson, D. (1987) Family status and health behaviour, social control as a dimension of social integration. *Journal of Health and Social Behaviour*, **28**, 306–19.

Varney Burst, H. (1983) The influence of consumers in the birthing movement. *Topics in Clinical Nursing*, **5**, 42–54.

Vehviläinen-Julkunen, K. & Liukkonen, A. (1998) Fathers' experiences of birth. *Midwifery*, **14**(1) 10–17.

Waldenström, U. (1998) Continuity of carer. *Midwifery*, **14**(4) 207–13.

Walker, J. (1976) Midwife or obstetric nurse? Some perceptions of midwives and obstetricians of the role of the midwife. *Journal of Advanced Nursing*, **1**, 129–138.

Walsh, D. (1996) Editorial: Evidence-based practice: whose evidence and on what basis? *British Journal of Midwifery*, **4**(9) 454–7.

Walsh, D. (1999) Demystifying clinical audit. *MIDIRS Midwifery Digest*, **9**(4) 430–1.

Walsh, F. (1989) The family in later life. Chapter 14, pp.311–32 in *The Changing Family Life Cycle* (eds B. Carter & M. McGoldrick) 2nd edn. Boston, Allyn & Bacon.

Walton, D., Field, R., McAdam, E., Derman, J., Gordon, N., Gallitero, G., Garrett, L. & Klaus, M. (1998) *The impact of a hospital based doula program in a health maintenance organization setting*. 18th Annual meeting of the Society of perinatal obstetricians, Florida.

Warwick, C.L. (1996) Supervision and Practice Change at Kings. Chapter 8, p.102 in *Supervision of Midwives* (ed. M. Kirkham). Hale, Books for Midwives Press.

Watkins, T.M. (1998) Defining women's preferences for support during labour: a review of the literature. *Journal of Perinatal Education*, **7**(4) 9–16.

Weaver, J. (1998) Choice, control and decision-making in labour. Chapter 5 in *Psychological Perspectives on Pregnancy and Childbirth* (ed. S. Clement). Edinburgh, Churchill Livingstone.

Webster, C. (2000) The early NHS and the crisis in public health nursing. *International History of Nursing Journal*, **5**(2) 4–10.

Webster, J., Linnane, J.W.J., Dibley, L.M., Hinson, J.K., Starrenburg, S.E. & Roberts, J.A. (2000) Measuring social support in Pregnancy: can it be simple and meaningful? *Birth*, **27**(2) 97–101.

Webster, J., Lloyd, W.C., Pritchard, M.A., Burridge, C.A., Plucknett, L.E. & Byrne, A.J. (1999) Development of evidence-based guidelines in midwifery and gynaecology nursing. *Midwifery*, **15**(1) 2–5.

Wessely, S. (1998) Commentary: Reducing distress after normal childbirth. *Birth*, **25**(4) 220–1.

Wessely, S., Rose, S. & Bisson, J. (2000) Brief psychological interventions ('debriefing') for trauma-related symptoms and the prevention of post traumatic stress disorder. *The Cochrane Database of Systematic Reviews*, (issue 1). The Cochrane Library, The Cochrane Collaboration.

Wheatley, S. (1998) Psychosocial support in pregnancy. Chapter 3, pp. 45–59 in *Psychological Perspectives on Pregnancy and Childbirth* (ed. S. Clement). Edinburgh, Churchill Livingstone.

Whelan, A. Lupton, P. (1998) Promoting successful breast feeding among women with a low income. *Midwifery*, **14**(2) 94–100.

WHO (1978) Alma Ata: *Report of the International Conference on Primary Health Care*. Geneva, World Health Organisation.

WHO (1985) World Health Organisation: appropriate technology for birth. *Lancet*, ii, (8452) 24 Aug, 436–7.

WHO (1986) *World Health Organisation Planning and Management for Health Report on a European Conference*. The Hague, WHO Regional Office for Europe.

WHO/UNICEF (1989) *Protecting promoting and supporting breastfeeding: The Special Role of Maternity Services*. A joint WHO/UNICEF statement. Geneva, World Health Organisation.

Wiegers, T.A., Keirse, M.J., Berghs, G.A. & van der Zee, J. (1996) An approach to measuring quality of midwifery care. *Journal of Clinical Epidemiology*, **49**(3) 319–25.

Wills, T.A. (1985) Supportive functions of interpersonal relationships. Chapter 4, pp.61–82 in *Social Support and Health* (S. Cohen & S.L. Syme). Orlando, Academic Press.

Winterton Report (1992) House of Commons Health Committee Second Report. *Maternity Services*, vol. 1. London, The Stationery Office.

Wraight, A., Ball, J., Seccombe, I. & Stock, J. (1993) *Mapping team midwifery*. Brington, Institute of Manpower Studies.

Young, D. (1998) Doulas: into the mainstream of maternity care. *Birth*, **25**(4) 213–14.

Young, G. (1999) The case for community-based maternity care. Chapter 2, pp.7–26 in *Community-based Maternity Care* (eds G. Marsh & M. Renfrew). General Practice Series, Oxford University Press.

Index